What Am I Thinking?

What Am I Thinking?

Having a Baby After Postpartum Depression

*What you've been through, what you have learned,
and what you still need to know*

KAREN KLEIMAN, MSW

Author of *The Postpartum Husband* and co-author of *This Isn't What I Expected*

To order additional copies of this book, contact:
Xlibris Corporation
1-888-795-4274
www.Xlibris.com
Orders@Xlibris.com
26124

CONTENTS

Section Four
Preparing For Pregnancy And Another Baby

For Jeff and Melanie,
who continue to inspire my work,
my life, my heart and my soul.

Foreword

Many women and their partners enter childbearing with a sense of how many children to have. For some it's an approximate number: let's have a couple and decide if we want a third later. For some it's highly specific: we had four children in my family and that's exactly what I want. Many factors go into deciding family size. Some have a religious orientation that supports large families, others have economic circumstances that limit family size. Nature or fate may determine it: the couple planning on having an only child finds that a certain romantic evening has altered their plans. Others want a mixed family, and will try once or twice more to get that daughter or son that hasn't yet appeared.

Postpartum depression trumps most if not all other considerations. The first time it hits a family, it is virtually always unexpected. Who could imagine that a wanted, loved baby could be accompanied by such significant pain and distress? Until the woman suffering from postpartum depression (or OCD, anxiety, or psychosis) experiences it herself, she may have believed any or all of the myths of blissful motherhood, or thought that postpartum disorders were rare, something that happened to crazy ladies on television.

But once it hits home, you know better. You know that a mother who welcomes motherhood, loves her baby, and is emotionally ready for parenthood may not have the brain chemistry to sustain her through this vulnerable time. Or, you may learn first hand that postpartum depression, while controlled or seemingly "cured" by medication and/or therapy, can linger, and make it difficult to feel well without ongoing treatment. And that means that the second, or third, or fourth baby, the one you always planned on having, isn't so simple. Whatever your original plan was, you now know something that you didn't know before: the postpartum period can be horrendous. Your odds of another bout are much higher than other women's risk, and you yourself know how bad a bad PPD can be.

But you want another baby. Or maybe you do, if you can improve your odds of an easier transition following the next childbirth. Or maybe your husband does, and you need to help him understand why you want to stop with the family size you have. Or maybe he thinks only a masochist would risk another bout of PPD, and you want to let him know why you think having another baby is worth the risk.

Karen Kleiman's book addresses the questions that mothers want asked. Should postpartum depression prevent you from having the family size you always wanted? Would a loving mother risk another bout—how would that affect her other children? Her husband? Can you prevent it? Can you do things to reduce your risk, or make it less devastating if you get a second bout of PPD? Will medication help? How can you stress-proof your life, knowing what you know this time? In the worst case scenario, does early diagnosis and intervention facilitate a more rapid recovery?

This book is packed with information to help the woman, and her partner, make the best decision for herself and her family. Karen's vast clinical experience working with women across the spectrum of postpartum disorders—and their families—puts her in a unique position to address the complexities of the decision. Along with information, Karen provides the emotional support and guidance that women grappling with the decision whether to risk another bout of PPD need. *What Am I Thinking: Having a Baby After Postpartum Depression* will be an enormously useful and sensitive companion for anyone facing one of the most gut-wrenching decisions a woman will ever make.

Valerie Davis Raskin, MD,
Author of "*When Words Are Not Enough*"

Prologue

One woman contemplates her baby's demise. Another one has her name splashed all over the newspapers detailing the gruesome and deliberate manner in which she *saved her children from their fate on earth by helping them find their way to heaven.* And still another leaps to her death leaving a note behind reminding her loved ones that their lives will be fuller without her here.

The stories are unimaginable and horrific. The epitome of something gone terribly wrong? A diagnosis missed? A family adrift? A disease out-of-control?

Accounts similar to these have recently gripped the headlines and more and more women with postpartum depression have found themselves trying to deal with disheartening new and unspoken fears. *Will I, too, act on some of my deepest, darkest, most secret thoughts that somehow bring harm to my baby? What if I become psychotic? What will happen if I tell someone how I'm really feeling?*

After recent tragedies hit far too close to home and the predictable media frenzy that ensued, I was contacted by a number of reporters who tried to make sense out of it all: "Well, let's hope some good can come out of this," one journalist optimistically declared. "Maybe this will make it easier for women to come forward and talk about how they're feeling so they can get help."

Maybe.

But that's not what's happening. Women are more afraid than ever.

Women are afraid that they will totally lose control. They are frightened that the healthcare system won't understand, or worse, will betray them. They are frightened that they must continue to suffer in silence because the risk of disclosure is way too high. Perhaps worst of all, they remain terrified of their own thoughts, their paralyzing feelings, and most afraid of the deep despair that lurks behind the face they put on to get them through each day when they are suffering from PPD.

And the pretense persists. Women remain imprisoned by their fears, afraid to move forward, and at the same time, they must try to present a picture of total control to everyone around them. The illusion of control is vital. This is partly so they can convince themselves that they are okay and partly so they can convince everyone else. Claire described it this way, "I wish I felt as good as I look like I feel."

If you ask a woman who has never had a baby if she's worried about postpartum depression, she is likely to say it probably won't happen to her. If you ask a woman who is currently depressed how she feels about having another baby, she will likely say she will never have any more children. If you ask a woman who has recovered from postpartum depression how she feels about having another baby, she is likely to say she is afraid. One of the first questions women ask me when they come into my office is "Did you have postpartum depression?" I have mixed feelings, thinking I am both disappointing them and reassuring them as mothers when I respond, "No, I did not." When I co-authored my first book, *This Isn't What I Expected* with Valerie Davis Raskin, MD, we both remarked about the depth of the information we had been taught by our clients. It was, indeed, the information clients shared with us that enabled us to help them—because no matter how skilled and educated and well-trained I claimed or hoped to be, I had not known, not *really* known, the depths of despair that can descend upon the soul of a mother. I had not really known the shame and the agony of not loving your baby, or loving your baby too much, or not trusting your instincts or thinking your family would be better off if you were gone. I had not really known how hard it can be to simply get through the day when every effort feels impossible and every breath hurts.

But now I do know. I know because of the extraordinary women who have trusted me enough to share their deeply private thoughts and made the journey, with me, through the pain and back into the light. It's a remarkable journey, really. To say that I enjoy it would sound too dismissive or cavalier, if not out-and-out disrespectful to these women and to their traumas. But I haven't found the right words to describe how inspiring it feels for me to talk with someone who believes in the power of our relationship and the difference it can make in their lives. I have seen women inch their way up from the deepest abyss, steadfast in their conviction that life has no meaning and it really doesn't matter to them whether they live or not, and then, like a miracle, rise again to face another day with renewed hope and joy in their hearts. It's an experience I never take for granted. And so, again, I find myself turning to the women who continue to shape the work that I do. Here's what many are saying now: They're telling me how much they've been through, how strong they feel for the most part and how terrified they feel about having another baby. It's that clear. In some ways, it's very black and white to these moms. *I've had a baby. I've endured and survived the agony of postpartum depression. I'm thinking of having another baby. I am petrified of going through that again. I don't know what to do.*

Women decide to have or to *not* have another baby for a variety of reasons. For you who decide to go forward with another pregnancy after postpartum depression, the path from a previous experience with depression to the unknown events that surround another pregnancy can feel insurmountable. My purpose in this book is to make this next journey a bit less scary for you, to arm you with information and the confidence to know you are moving in the direction that is best for you, and to support your own ability to make a choice that is right for you and your family.

If you have a history of postpartum depression, you know how overwhelming the thought of having another baby is. Though the majority of this book is geared toward the woman's experience of depression and motherhood (simply because it is my assumption that women are more likely to be reading the book than their husbands/spouses/partners, at least at first!), it goes without saying that partners are an equal part of this picture. It is my hope that as a couple, the two of you will share what you learn in this book, supporting each other and using your reading and discussion as continuing opportunities to express your concerns and to get things out in the open. Straightforward communication will ease your anxieties and set the groundwork in motion to insure a smoother and more meaningful experience for you and your family.

There is no doubt in my mind that the more knowledge you have, the less you will fear the unknown. Making sure you feel in control of this situation is my primary objective. Therefore, as a result of the work that I do and the guiding words of the women I speak with every day, the information in this book will help relieve your apprehensions and strengthen your resolve as you move forward in this process.

Our work in this book will weave together the following concepts: Making sure you understand what postpartum depression is, what your personal experience with it was in the past, and how that impacted your life, your marriage, your family, your spirit, and making sure that what we do to prepare for the next pregnancy will make you feel strong and hopeful and certainly, less afraid. Keep in mind that all the hard work you do while you are struggling with the concepts in this book will be most helpful in conjunction with the work you do with your therapist and your doctor so that you can promote communication among your healthcare practitioners. If you don't have a therapist and think one would be helpful, ask your healthcare practitioner for a referral. In addition to the support and guidance they offer you, this book and the worksheets included will provide valuable information for the team of professionals supporting you. Share your work with them. Remember that my words, the voice and experience of the women who helped shape this book, and your belief in yourself will work together to maintain your strength and stability on the uncertain path that lies ahead. You don't have to go through this alone. There are answers to your questions, there is information that will validate your concerns and guide you in the right direction. The experience of another pregnancy can truly be something to anticipate with desire and not fear. I hope to help you make that happen for you.

Karen Kleiman, MSW

Introduction

Women's Voices

What follows is a sample of women's responses to a questionnaire for women at The Postpartum Stress Center who were thinking about having another baby after PPD. The words are their own, written anonymously in response to the questions below.

WHAT WORRIES YOU RIGHT NOW?

"Do I really want to go through this again? What if it is worse this time? What if I can't take care of the baby again but now there are other kids? Will I hurt them if it gets worse?"

"Being on medication during pregnancy. I don't want to stop the medication because I am terrified of feeling awful again but I don't want to hurt my baby either."

"Relapse. Also I worry about the health of our next baby. Even though I think my antidepressant is safe based on the anecdotal evidence."

"The occasional physical symptoms I still have, despite being on my way to recovery from PPD. How much longer will I need to be on medication and what will happen when I go off it?"

"The last trimester/month—possible sleep apnea and panic attacks— and associated depression. Delivery—another possible C-section."

"That my depression will be worse this time and I won't be able to take care of the baby. That things will get totally out of control."

WHAT WOULD HELP YOU THE MOST RIGHT NOW?

"A plan. An outline of what I need to do and when."

"Continuing therapy and learning more about PPD."

"Support group. Clear studies on medications and pregnancy or at least a gathering as much data from women who have had babies with and without meds."

"Being able to not have to think about PPD, which is starting to happen more often."

"A good support system in place prior to the last month and delivery."

"Just knowing that I've taken steps to do all the right things to take care of myself and my family will help. Staying connected with professionals who are familiar with my situation."

HOW DOES YOUR HUSBAND FEEL ABOUT ALL OF THIS?

"Not sure if he wants to go through it again. He's very concerned for my safety."

"He is ready to start again and encourages me to be excited. He says we can deal with anything I might go through after what we've been through."

"He is supportive and we are in agreement about our plans for my second pregnancy and child. I know he is concerned about relapse. He doesn't want to see me go through that again!"

"He is not concerned about having a second child as my PPD was not severe and I've responded well to treatment."

"Extremely supportive, but worried that he won't be able to do as much this time around due to his work schedule."

"He's nervous, mostly because I'm nervous, I think."

WHAT IS YOUR SINGLE GREATEST FEAR?

"If I could hurt the kids if this gets worse and how bad it will get."

"Feeling terrible again."
"Being so depressed that I harm my children emotionally or physically."

"A recurrence of pre-eclampsia and the effects it could have on my and the baby's health."

"That I will 'lose it' after the baby's born. That it will be so overwhelming and terrible. That my mother will be unsupportive."

"That I will never get better, if I get sick again."

WHAT IS YOUR CURRENT PLAN REGARDING MEDICATION?

"Continue meds until it's okay to come off. Doctor said I could continue the antidepressant into pregnancy if need be or start it at the end of the pregnancy, whatever I need."

"Staying on it!!"

"I'm currently taking 100mg of my antidepressant every day. I don't plan on going off medication during pregnancy or while nursing because I suffered from depression before I was pregnant and then later again. I've had it all my life on and off. The risk of my going into a deep depression is greater for me than my baby's exposure to my small dose of antidepressant."

"I am hoping I will not need medication until postpartum, if at all."

"I'm currently on 40mg of my antidepressant and that's the plan as far as I know. During pregnancy and after. But we'll see."

"Before my last PPD, I would have sworn I would NEVER take meds. Now, after what I went through, I am ready to pop that pill in my mouth as soon as this baby comes out!"

ANYTHING ELSE YOU WOULD LIKE US TO KNOW?

"There is so much fear. Before we only worried about money before making a decision to have another baby. Now, I'm really scared about me."

"I am actually less scared about going through an ordeal again because now my husband and I are aware of what to look for."

"Therapy and medication saved my life. When I returned to work and my son was 6 months old I became more depressed than I'd ever been in my life. I'm working full time again a year later and although I don't like it and it's stressful, I'm not in a crisis situation about it. I had only done therapy in the past. This is my first time using medication for my depression and I'm glad I did!"

Section One

FEAR

What if I get depressed again?

- *What if I can't function?*
- *What if my depression gets so bad I can't get out of bed or do anything?*
- *How will I take care of my baby?*
- *How will I take care of my older child?*
- *What if it's even worse this time?*
- *What if I do something horrible?*
- *What if I'm making a terrible mistake?*

Of course you're worried about having another baby. This is a good thing. It is an indication you will work hard to prepare the groundwork for this event. I am far more concerned about women who have experienced a severe depression in the past and are *not* worried about this occurring again. Jackie was eight months postpartum and seven months post-hospitalization. The treatment she received after her overdose of sleeping pills had successfully brought her back to herself, she was healthy again, bursting with love and deep pleasure from her son whom she often referred to as "the love of my life." When she came into my office one day, she sat down full of strength and beaming with exuberance. She turned to me with a meaningful smile and lifted brows that seemed to await my response. "Guess what? . . . I'm pregnant!" she blurted out, too eager to pause for my response.

This was not what I expected to hear. It wasn't only that she announced she was pregnant at a time that I thought would be clinically premature. It was more her sheer euphoria. It was her apparent lack of concern for her recent and quite severe postpartum depression and the implications of her past experience for another pregnancy. It was, perhaps, the fact that I was the only one in that room who felt uneasy about this prospect. Jackie's dismissal of her recent crisis is not typical of what I see in my practice. It is, however, of great concern to me, which is why I mention it here.

In contrast to the majority of women who are terrified of getting pregnant again after PPD, women who protect themselves by suppressing their traumatic memories, though more likely to feel better in the short run, run the risk of critically interfering with their ability to prepare for the immense vulnerability to PPD that can return again. Therefore it bears repeating, it's *good* that you're worried about getting depressed again. You may not get depressed again this time. But you might. And you are far better off if you prepare for that possibility.

♦

Experts are often asked *what's the difference between postpartum depression and "regular" depression, that is, depression that is not related to childbirth?* The answer is not so simple. Postpartum depression is the presence of a clinical depression after the birth of a child (usually within the first year). In this way, PPD is just like any other clinical depression. The symptoms are often the same. The treatment is often the same.

However, in order for PPD to be entirely understood and properly treated, it needs to be understood within the context of having a baby. In other words, in addition to feeling sad, hopeless, frightened, and unable to think clearly, *there is another tiny person, a new baby, in the picture.* This means that on top of the depressive symptoms, women are also forced to cope with sleep deprivation, hormonal vulnerabilities, transition from being a pregnant woman to the role of being the mother of a newborn, leaky breasts or 3 a.m. formula recipes, as well as the demanding recovery from the childbirth experience itself, and don't forget, there is already a child to be taken care of and loved, as well as a partner who has already been through this process once and may not be feeling all that confident of his ability to do it again.

Under ideal circumstances and in most situations, no one expects to get depressed after having a baby. Most women and their families expect this will be *the happiest time of their lives.* We've all heard that before. The expectations that accompany this notion are that good mothers experience and embrace the joy and contentment that naturally follow childbirth. Therefore, a woman who becomes depressed after childbirth has been thrust into motherhood with sudden reversals of expectations and without the emotional foundation she thought she would have to sustain her. So the drama unfolds and the cycle begins anew. Symptoms emerge and guilt sets in. Her feelings of inadequacy swell as she begins to realize that she is probably not going to be able to function the way she had hoped she was going to be capable of. The less she does, the worse she feels. The worse she feels, the less she can do. Her dependency alarms her and her failure to "do this right" might even enrage her at times. Yet, she cannot rise above the dark cloud. And so she sinks.

When we look closely at this picture, as bad as it might make you feel when you read it or think about it, it's important to keep this image in mind when you review your options about having another baby. The last thing I want to do is make this more complicated for you. But believe me when I tell you that if we don't get down and dirty and examine all the things you are truly most afraid of, you will not be able to proceed in this decision-making process with confidence and the belief that you are doing the right thing. Why are we doing this? Why are you so concerned and why am I so interested in addressing your concerns? Because the bottom line is this: *If you've had postpartum depression once before, you are at risk of having it again and if you are not properly treated, the depression can be worse the second time.* This is why we are going to make sure we cover all the bases so you and your partner and family are comfortable with your conclusions and can make this important decision with confidence.

It's hard enough to have a baby when you're feeling good. The demands on your body, your mind, and your spirit are huge. It's not surprising, therefore, that any compromise in your physical, mental, and emotional state will make everything that much harder.

Robin lies in bed after another sleepless night. She can't decide which feels worse, lying there, bombarded by anxious thoughts of how she will get through the day, or mustering up the energy to get out of bed to face another endless day she feels she will not be able to endure. Each morning is the same. She can't breathe, though she knows she must be breathing because her heart is racing so hard she can feel it pounding through her chest. It's all she can think about, how bad she feels, how inadequate she must be, how guilty this makes her, how this will only get worse, how she will always feel this way and never get better, how no one understands how bad she feels. Her mind won't turn off. "How can I possibly get through another day feeling like this," she thinks. Then, when she finally convinces herself it's okay to close her eyes and rest her weary brain, she thinks about her baby and a shock wave stuns her from the outside in. She lies motionless, unable to either rest comfortably or move forward.

Robin's depression is awful enough to think about. But if we add another child to that scenario and envision a toddler in the background also needing Mom's attention, the paralysis becomes even more intense. Imagine that this toddler is the one who was there navigating the rough terrain of PPD with her. Imagine further, that after everything they went through together, her greatest desire, even stronger than her desire to be there for her new baby, is that her older child never *ever* experiences that disconnect again.

◆

Depression is more than a bad mood. It's more than a string of cranky days that make you feel like you want to crawl out of your own skin. It's more than a persistent negative attitude. Depression is an illness that can take over your entire body. It involves your mind, your spirit, your brain chemistry, your heredity, your living situation and environment, your current stressors, your history, and your expectations. It affects the way you think, the way you feel, and the way you act. It's a medical condition that requires and responds to medical treatment. If not treated properly, it can linger or it can get worse.

The good news about depression is that in many cases, it can speak on your behalf. Sometimes, the symptoms serve as a valuable means to an end. That is, if you listen to what the symptoms are telling you, you may have a better understanding of how best to intervene with any subsequent depression as well as gain a deeper understanding of who you are and what you need. As an example of this, consider the need to be cared for and to be nurtured during the postpartum period. Carly describes it like this:

"All my life I felt like my mother wasn't there for me. She was busy or distracted. She tried, I know she tried, but she worked a lot after the divorce and just couldn't be there. When I got married and moved away, it was hard for me to be on my own, even though I knew it was expected of me. And then I had the baby and everything fell apart. I tried so hard not to turn to my mother. I thought that would just prove what a bad mother I was and what a baby I still was and that I'd never be able to do this by myself. So I toughed it out for a while, but then my symptoms got worse. It was like, the harder I tried, the sicker I got. When things got unbearable, my husband called my mother and asked if she'd make the trip to spend some time here with me. She did. It was wonderful. When I finally gave myself permission to let her take care of me this way, it felt so good."

The needs of postpartum women are uniquely complicated. They range from the physical and hormonal to the emotional and spiritual. As we saw with Carly, specific emotional needs can come to the surface, sometimes for the first time, during the postpartum period, which is the time in a woman's life when she is most vulnerable to emotional illness.

Each of you has areas of vulnerability and needs that may not be met as adequately as you might like. But you do what you have to do to compensate, you get through the day just fine, you "keep on keepin' on" armed with your coping mechanisms and for the most part, you are very successful at all of this.

And then, you have a baby. You become sleep deprived, hormonally compromised, irritable and anxious, and all of a sudden, everything you have ever known that made sense is upside down. You work hard to keep up appearances, but the personal resources you rely on from day to day are dwindling. Your needs shift dramatically from being the one who kept everything under control and took care of everything to being the one who requires a certain amount of caretaking. Many women with babies reveal a secret and usually temporary desire to be mothered during this time period. This expression of dependency is perfectly normal and can be expected, although a desire for mothering for herself can be perceived by a woman as a negative, a regression that she is not prepared to accept. Embracing and exploring this desire to be cared for (either by your own mother, a mother-figure, or another loving caretaker, such as your partner) could be a very interesting pathway to explore in preparation for another pregnancy.

What if I get anxious again?

Elise spent hours wondering if she should take her baby to the doctor. After a two-week treatment with antibiotics for an ear infection, her five-month old daughter was given a clean bill of health by the pediatrician. But Elise couldn't help worrying, "what if the doctor was wrong? What if he missed something?" If she brought her baby out to the mall, would she get sick again? What if someone who was sick touched her baby? How could she make certain that she would be protected? Elise was always a worrier. But now it seemed so much worse. Before, she would worry about simple things, like what time to leave for an appointment so she could avoid the traffic and not be late, or she'd worry about losing her job if she wasn't working hard enough. Sometimes, she worries about whether she and her husband will be able to afford the house she wants.

Now, Elise's worry has taken on new forms. She worries that someone will break into the house and take her baby, or worse, kill her baby. She worries she might accidentally drop the baby or make the bath water too hot and scald her. She worries about the amount of food she's giving her, the number of naps her daughter's taking, the diaper rash that doesn't seem to go away and she worries about whether her baby girl will have good friends and go to college.

Will you get anxious again? Unequivocally yes. You will. Most definitely. In fact, you will get anxious again whether you decide to have another baby or not. It's one of the only absolutes in this book. Anxiety and motherhood go hand in hand. It's not possible to be good mothers without worrying about how life impacts your babies and how the choices you make influence everything else along the way. What an awesome responsibility! Welcome to the world of motherhood, the good, the bad, and the ugly, to be sure.

Accepting a certain amount of anxiety is not only a healthy response, it provides you with the tools to cope with the anxiety that feels out of your control from time to time.

If anxiety becomes excessive, that is, if it interferes with your ability to experience pleasure, or if it becomes the focus of your day, then that's too much anxiety and that's no longer okay. This is when you need to follow up with a professional or with an intervention that has helped you in the past.

If anxiety is experienced as extremely problematic (that is, if it feels like it's wrong or bad to have any anxiety at all, especially about being a mom), the more likely you are to feel threatened and the worse you will feel. In other words, if we assume that anxiety is present and we accept this in many situations, then it is the *degree* of anxiety that makes a difference in terms of the person's experience. The last thing we want to do is to *worry about the worrying*, which is guaranteed to intensify the anxiety.

Laurie was also a worrier. After her baby was born, her worry took on new dimensions. *All new moms worry*, she would think. Did the baby have enough to eat? What if the baby missed her nap? What if she gets exposed to someone's cold if they go the shopping center? Or worse, what if something terrible happens while they're out? Will she be safe in the car? Laurie could hear her worrying thoughts spinning around in her head. *Uh-oh, this isn't good. Why am I thinking these things? Does this mean something bad IS going to happen? Is it normal to worry like this? Maybe something else is wrong with me. Is this what happens when mothers hurt their babies? Is that why my head is so cluttered with worry?*

Laurie is quite right about one thing. It is normal for mothers to worry about their babies. Anxiety is an exaggeration of a normal healthy response. That's why it can be hard to distinguish, sometimes. If all mothers worry, to some extent, how does one know how much worrying is okay? When does it become a problem? As you probably know from your own experience, worry and anxiety can take on a life of their own, it can feed itself and grow larger and more troublesome. You and your worrying thoughts can slide down that slippery slope without you really knowing what's happening until you find yourself consumed by agonizing anxiety.

One of the most powerful ways for you to manage your anxiety is to begin with the understanding that some degree of anxiety is to be expected. For example, it's perfectly fine for you to worry about the timing of your baby's nap or whether she's warm enough. These are instincts that will insure your baby's well-being and comfort. What we do *not* want, however, is for this worry to interfere with your ability to get through the day. Frankly, some women can operate very well with high degrees of anxiety, while others find it gets in the way of optimal functioning very quickly. If we accept the fact that anxiety will be present, we will have more control over its impact.

One of the best ways to achieve this sense of control is to realize that you have more power over your anxiety than you might think you have. Women in my office are quite familiar with my reference to a scale of anxiety tolerance. "On a scale of 0-10, how high is your anxiety right now?" is something they hear me say on a regular basis. It's an anxiety check. That's because anxiety is fluid, it can go up and down, back and forth, better or worse, any time of day or night.

You cannot always control the events that triggered the original anxiety, but you can control how you respond to the anxiety and do things to make it better or worse. You can, for instance, learn how to move it from a 7 down to a 6 or from a 9 to an 8. Some people find relaxation or breathing exercises helpful to accomplish this. Other people prefer to use distraction techniques. The trick is to understand and expect that anxiety will be there, but watch it move up and hopefully down, so *you* can be the one controlling it, rather than it controlling you. Any incremental change you can make or power you can claim over your anxiety is terrific. Belief in your ability to adjust the anxiety even a little bit can bring enormous relief.

The key here is to be able to figure out what degree of anxiety falls within normal limits and how much is too much. That's not always an easy distinction to make, not for anyone, but certainly not for someone who's hyperfocusing on how they feel or is super sensitive to anxiety in the first place. If you are ever not sure whether what you are feeling is okay or not, that's a good enough reason to check with your healthcare provider or therapist to get some perspective on your emotional state.

Worst case scenario

What's your greatest fear right now? When asked, most women say they are afraid their illness will be worse the next time. "*What if next time I do something that hurts my baby?*" or "*What if next time I end up like those women on T.V.?*"

Think about what you are most afraid of. Sometimes, by laying it all out up front, it makes it real, it makes the fear something you can potentially deal with, it makes it smaller and more manageable than the hold it has on you when it's a private, unspoken fear.

- ❏ I'm afraid my depression will be worse this time.
- ❏ I'm afraid I will really go crazy.
- ❏ I wonder if I even had postpartum depression in the first place.
- ❏ I wonder if I had the best treatment and why it took so long for me to feel better.

❑ What if I get an illness that's different this time and harder to treat and I never get better?

❑ I don't think I can go through this again alone. I don't have enough help.

❑ Even the thought of getting pregnant again terrifies me.

❑ What if the medication doesn't work this time?

❑ What if my symptoms return while I'm pregnant?

❑ What can I do to make sure this doesn't happen again?

❑ What if my partner can't handle this again?

❑ What if my partner didn't handle it so well the first time?

❑ What if I hurt my baby?

❑ What about medication? Should I stop the medication I'm taking if I find out I'm pregnant? If I start medication while I'm pregnant, will it prevent PPD? Can I take medication if I breastfeed?

Think about your worst case scenario. The depression returns. Symptoms resurface. Chances are if you do experience depression this time around, you will have an illness similar to your previous one, not worse. If you're worried about postpartum psychosis, remember that depression and psychosis are two distinct illnesses, one does not turn into the other.

Keep this in mind:

• Here are some terms you should be familiar with:

    Unipolar depression is a major depression without mania. Basically, this would be any major depression that is not bipolar.

    Bipolar depression, also known as manic-depression, is characterized by moods that swing between two opposite poles, mania or extreme elation and depression

    Psychosis refers to a severe mental disorder marked by extreme impairment of a person's ability to think clearly, respond or behave appropriately, and understand reality.

    Obsessive-compulsive Disorder (OCD) is an illness that causes unwanted, intrusive thoughts often associated with the urge to repeat certain behaviors over and over again.

- If you have been treated for a unipolar depression, you are at risk for *depression* again, *not psychosis.*
- If you had postpartum psychosis, you are at risk for psychosis after another pregnancy.
- If you have been treated for bipolar disorder in the past, or schizophrenia, you are at risk for psychosis.
- If a close blood relative has been treated for bipolar disorder or schizophrenia, your risk for psychosis after childbirth increases.

For the most part, the fear of getting postpartum psychosis is an irrational fear, not based in reality. It is based on an unfounded although understandable fear which is often the result of sensationalized media attention following a tragedy of unthinkable proportions. The only advantage worrying about your worst case scenario can have is that it will help you prepare. Women who prepare are not the women who are blindsided by an illness out of control. *No matter what your previous diagnosis was or what your treatment consisted of or what you are afraid will happen next time, early intervention makes all the difference.* Early intervention refers to getting a proper diagnosis with appropriate treatment and follow-up. Having a plan, mobilizing your resources, and getting everyone and everything on board for the event will significantly increase the likelihood that if you do experience problems, your symptoms will respond well and quickly to treatment.

What if I really go crazy this time?

What if anxiety gets the better of you? What if for an instant all your anxious and distorted thoughts became real? What if these thoughts were no longer merely figments of your imagination? What if they were not over-exaggerated neurotic interpretations as your loving family once reassured you? What if for one excruciating moment in time, everything you ever feared the most was realized? What if you could no longer distinguish between what you really needed to be afraid of and what was only a daydream or a nightmare? What if all boundaries got blurred and nothing made sense anymore? And perhaps worst of all, what if you *knew* nothing was making sense? Almost as if there was a part of your mind that was outside watching how crazy you felt inside?

Awful scenario.

The truth is, this is how acute anxiety can make you feel. Anxiety? If you've experienced this, you know very well what I'm talking about. If you have not, you might be surprised to learn how unbelievably brutal the experience of severe anxiety can be. And yes, it can feel like you're going crazy.

Jody was four months postpartum when she described the panic that grabbed her out of nowhere:

I was just walking in the mall, minding my own business. I knew I wasn't feeling good, things just weren't right. I had been planning to call my doctor for a few days and honestly, I hoped things would just get better if I stopped thinking about it. I mean, I was nervous and felt shaky but I didn't think anything horrible was happening. But when the saleswoman asked for my money, I had no idea what she was saying or how to respond. I could feel the line of people behind me breathing down my back, waiting for me to do something, say something, or at least, get out of the way. I couldn't move. It was like I was in slow motion and everything else was racing around me. My thoughts were darting from corner to corner of my mind while my body stood frozen. I felt sick to my stomach and my hearted pounded out of my chest. I couldn't think, I couldn't breathe. I wanted to scream but couldn't move. I felt like I was separate from my body as if I had no control over what was happening to me. The more I tried to focus, the more I panicked. Something horrible was happening, but I didn't know what. I have no idea how long I was standing there. As if on auto pilot, I paid the woman and escorted my numb self out of the store. I sat in my car crying, wondering if I should drive myself to the emergency room or just sit there forever. I couldn't believe how out of it I felt.

Jody didn't go crazy. But she felt as if she had. And thought, for sure, it would happen the "next" time.

Anxiety is a dreadful beast. It can cause constant, unremitting terror that permeates a person's day. It can play tricks with your mind, it can make things feel unreal, and it can make you question things you have always known to be true. We all have habits in our daily lives or routines that we like to do over and over the same way. But people with obsessive compulsive tendencies may demonstrate patterns of behavior that get in the way of their daily life or stop them from doing certain things due to intense fear or anxiety. If you have obsessive-compulsive symptoms it can feel like you can't control the thoughts and behaviors that accompany those thoughts. You might be plagued by invasive persistent thoughts or images that seem to dart out of nowhere.

Women with postpartum depression sometimes feel like they are going crazy. They are not. Postpartum depression frequently appears as a very agitated depression. This means that anxiety can be a predominant symptom and for some women, causes the most distress. Katherine Wisner, a leading researcher in postpartum depression, found women with PPD have increased rates of obsessional thoughts that are aggressive in nature compared to women with depression that is not linked to childbirth (Wisner, 1999). The presence of acute anxiety, depressive symptoms, and a new baby in the same picture can generate a wide range of unwelcome thoughts and feelings:

Why did I have this baby?
What if I do something to hurt my baby?
If he doesn't stop crying what if I do something awful, what if I can't help myself?
Why can't I get that image out of my head?
What if I drop the baby down the steps?
What if I burn the baby in the bathtub because I didn't test the water temperature properly?
What if I actually allow something horrible to happen because I honestly think my life was better before I had this baby?
What if I can no longer control these thoughts?
What if I really do something to hurt my baby, like burn her or cut her or abuse her?
What if I'm a terrible person and I accidentally or deliberately mistreat her or cause violent harm?
What if I can't endure the pain these thoughts are causing me?

Thoughts like these and others which can be extremely graphic and disturbing are more common than you might think with PPD. Women diagnosed with postpartum OCD can experience these kinds of thoughts quite regularly. Understanding what they are and just as importantly, what they are not, will provide you much needed relief. Simply put, they are symptoms of anxiety. They are *not* symptoms of psychosis.

Postpartum psychosis is very rare. It occurs in approximately one to two of every thousand new mothers. It is the most severe kind of postpartum disorder, requiring immediate and aggressive medical intervention, usually hospitalization. Studies have found more than half of all cases of postpartum psychosis begin in the first postpartum week and more than 75% occur within the first two weeks following delivery.

The severe symptoms usually begin abruptly and often include:

- Extreme confusion
- Hallucinations, hearing voices telling them to act in certain ways or seeing things that are unreal
- Delusions or false beliefs
- Hyperactivity and rapid speech
- Paranoia (unfounded distrust and suspicion)
- Changeable (labile) mood
- Frenzied energy, mania
- Severe depressive symptoms
- Suicidal and/or murderous (homicidal) thoughts that may be directed toward the baby

The list of symptoms can be intimidating, but it's important to be aware of them. Health professionals and family members also need to be on the lookout for the rapid onset of such severe symptoms such as these to avoid any delay in treatment. Women with postpartum psychosis might not realize they're having problems and may be unable or unwilling to seek treatment.

Women often tell me they are most fearful of "waking up psychotic" or fear they might suddenly feel compelled to follow imaginary commands to harm their babies, although they are having no such symptoms. Many women fear they will "snap" and do something that would bring harm to their babies, often avoiding contact with their babies to protect them from their irrational fear. But this isn't the way it happens and in fact, women who recognize these thoughts as irrational and are deeply disturbed by them are not psychotic.

Women with acute anxiety can experience negative intrusive thoughts, which often focus on harm coming to the baby. These thoughts come out of nowhere, make no sense, and are incredibly upsetting to women who struggle with this symptom. For women with postpartum OCD, these thoughts can be persistent, highly invasive, and round-the-clock. For women with PPD the impact of such thoughts may be equally distressing, although the thoughts themselves may be less severe or less prevalent.

These intrusive thoughts, associated with acute anxiety, are called "ego dystonic," meaning they are viewed as inconsistent with one's fundamental belief system and personality. That's what makes these thoughts so alarming to the mother experiencing them. That's also why it's a "good sign" when women find these kind of thoughts so distressing. It means they are thinking rationally, even if they are terrified. Women with postpartum psychosis, on the other hand, believe that their hallucinations and delusions are real. There is often no differentiation between their bizarre thoughts and what they believe to be their reality. That's an important distinction Although the media often misleadingly links the two together, postpartum psychosis and postpartum depression are two completely different illnesses. Postpartum psychosis is not a worsening case of postpartum depression; it's a totally distinct psychological disorder. In the most severe cases of postpartum depression, the concern is that a woman may harm *herself*, not her baby.

Therefore be assured that you are not going to go crazy. You might, however, get postpartum depression again. Then again, you might not. There are no guarantees. However, if you do experience postpartum depression next time, it may be different from your previous experience. It may be different because of the work you're doing now in preparation. The difference I refer to here does not necessarily refer to the specific symptoms or the course of illness itself. Rather, the distinction may be the in way you approach and interpret the symptoms and the experience as a result of the work you are doing here. Remember that many women report feeling unprepared for PPD—*my doctor didn't warn me, I didn't think this could happen to me*—so they were caught off guard. You are likely to feel less frightened and more in control of the symptoms and the experience as a whole by taking the time to prepare in this way.

Section Two

GAINING CONTROL

Reviewing your options

"A recent study reports that 32% of women who suffered an episode of postpartum depression dramatically changed their future childbearing plans, resorting to adoption, abortion, or in some cases even sterilization." (Stowe ZN, Nemeroff CB. 1995)

Jackie: Every time I heard his cry I wanted to jump out the window, I swear. Or run away. I couldn't stand to be in my own skin. It was as if my entire body was on fire. I couldn't breathe. *Just take the baby away*, I would think. Please God just let me sleep. It was like nothing else mattered.

Now I look at him and think, Oh my God, how could I ever have felt that way? Where did that time go? How do I get it back? It's almost as if it all happened to someone else, like it wasn't really me. How could I have those thoughts about my baby? About myself? Like the only way out of that pain was to sleep and never wake up. In some ways, it doesn't seem real to me. Still, it seems altogether too real, too scary, too unbelievable. And look at me now (*she puts her hand on her belly*) . . . about to do it all again. (*laughing uncomfortably*) WHAT AM I THINKING?

Therapist: Jackie, remember there are some things that are very different now. This next time, it will be different.

Jackie: I know that. That's what I'm banking on. Gary and I have been talking about that, all the ways it will be different.

Therapist: Tell me what you and Gary have been talking about.

Jackie: Well, this time I'm on medication, I have Dr.

M . . . who's keeping an eye on things, I have you, and
I have the experience of getting through the depression
last time, to draw upon. I'll be better prepared because
the nanny will be there and my mother-in-law will
stay over so I can get some sleep. Gary will be watching
over me like a hawk, so he'll be right on top of things,
I'm sure. I'll know, somewhere in my head, that even if
I do get sick again, I'll get out of it, just like the last
time. I'll have a better understanding of what's going
on, hopefully (*she smiles tentatively*).

I smile back at her. Knowing that she's right, all those things WILL
make a difference. Being on the medication, having a psychiatrist
and therapist who know exactly what to look for and how to treat
postpartum depression, having a husband who is extremely
supportive and having the history of a successful recovery will all
help Jackie this next time around.

But still, I can't help being distracted by my quiet thoughts of a
time not so long ago, about a year earlier, when Jackie was in quite
a different place. Jackie just wanted to sleep. *Please please someone
take the baby so I can sleep. I can't do this anymore. I don't want to do
this anymore. Take him away. Make him stop crying! PLEASE. Please
let me sleep.*

The bottle of Tylenol PM in the bathroom was the only thing keeping
her company, it was the only thing that could help her sleep. Her
husband was at work. Her two-month old baby was in the next
room, calling for his next feeding. *I'm so tired. I just want to sleep . . .*

Jackie awoke in the Intensive Care Unit struggling to make sense
out of the Resident's cautionary advice regarding acetaminophen
overdose and acute liver failure.

Jackie: So, what do you think? *She gazes down and embraces her
                 growing belly.* Think everything will be okay this time?

Therapist: I think we have some work to do.
Jackie: Yes we do.

You're thinking of having another baby. Or you're already pregnant, and wondering if this is a good idea. Or you're nervous about the prospect for one or another or many reasons. You might be remembering how quickly things became so complicated the last time when you were blindsided by postpartum depression. That doesn't feel very reassuring, does it?

And then you think about where you are now. And you're better. Much better. (Or at least most days you feel that way.) And you wonder, still. Should I do that again? Will I get postpartum depression again? Will it be worse this time? Can I go through that another time?

Elizabeth wondered about the same things:

I always knew I wanted three children. I grew up in a family with three kids, I had one brother and one sister. That's what I always envisioned for my own life with my partner. Mark, me, and our three little ones. I never considered that anything would get in the way of our life plan. When I got pregnant with Ethan, I knew everything was falling into place. I loved being pregnant. I loved imagining how our life would be, how fulfilled I would be as a mother, how my marriage would swell with joy and pride at the accomplishment of our life together. It was almost as if my life up to that point had been put on hold, anticipating the arrival of, yes, the best thing that would ever happen to me. And then, when Ethan was born, a cruel twist of fate took all that away from me. I was left with my beautiful healthy baby boy I always dreamed of, amidst a vacuum of meaninglessness and despair. The feelings of depression were dark and thick. I hardly recognized myself. I couldn't think. Nothing made sense. After months of treatment and an unpredictable course of recovery, I worked hard to find my core self again, to reclaim my sense of hope and comfort in the better days I prayed were still to come. And now that we are there, now that we truly

can breathe freely and deeply—we are thinking of doing this all again?
That's hard for me to believe. But it's true.

Why do you want to have another baby?

❑   Because I want my child to have a sibling
❑   Because I always wanted two or three or four (or more!) children
❑   Because I want to have a boy
❑   Because I want to have a girl
❑   Because my partner wants another baby
❑   Because I feel like it's the "right" thing to do
❑   Because I've always imagined myself with a certain number of children
❑   I'm not sure *why* I want to have another baby
❑   I'm not sure *if* I want to have another baby
❑   _____

The decision to have a baby, or another baby, is a very individual and personal choice. And it's never an easy one. For most couples, it is a decision that is met with a variety of questions, ambivalences, worries, and anxieties as well as eager anticipation.

Under ideal circumstances, the decision to have a baby requires a thoughtful dialogue between the two partners, with careful consideration of all relevant issues and any potential bumps in the road.

But if you've experienced postpartum depression, all of the standard concerns that couples have seem to pale in comparison to the thought process you are going through in your effort to come to a decision about another baby.

To put it simply: Why would someone *voluntarily* put themselves in a situation in which they could potentially feel out of control, overwhelmed with hopelessness and grief, immobilized by anxiety and fear, unable to think clearly, or plagued by an indescribable veil of deep sadness that feels as if it will never ever go away? Surely, no one would willingly put themselves in this position.

Or would they?

IMPORTANT FACTS YOU NEED TO KNOW:

- *Postpartum depression is a complex combination of biological, emotional, and behavioral changes. The exact cause of this condition is still unknown.* We can speculate as to the reasons why you got it last time or why you might be at risk to get it again, but frankly, we don't always know. Sometimes, women with many risk factors do not experience PPD and sometimes women with no known risk factors experience a full blown episode. That's why it's best to prepare for the possibility.

- *The postpartum period is a time of heightened risk for psychiatric illness.* (Nonacs R, Cohen L, Viguera A, Reminick A, Harlow B) Under these circumstances, it is prudent to maximize support and mobilize all resources during this time period. This includes practical interventions as well as all support networks, both personal and professional.

- *Up to 85% of women experience postpartum affective instability during the first couple of weeks, referred to as the Baby Blues.* (Pitt B. 1973).

- *Most women will experience some degree of emotional upheaval during the first couple of weeks after delivery.* This is normal. It can include periods of weepiness, anxiety, extreme fatigue, and sadness. Women can also experience worry and feelings of doubt that are very unsettling, but are quite typical of these first early days and weeks. However, if these feelings persist beyond the 2-3 weeks postpartum or if the feelings are experienced as extremely disturbing, we consider the possibility that depression may be setting in and further evaluation is indicated. Although baby blues is considered to be a typical reaction following childbirth, it is believed that mothers with severe baby blues are at high risk for depression (Beck *et al.* 1992).

- *Statistics seem to vary greatly, but it is generally agreed that postpartum depression occurs in 15-20% of women in the general population.* (Kumar & Robson 1984, Stein 1991, Cox et al. 1987, Jadresic 1995).
- *Postpartum depression can occur after the birth of any child, not just the first.* (ACOG Patient Education Pamphlet, 1990)
- *Women with prior history of depression or family history of a mood disorder are at increased risk for postpartum depression.* (Moline M, Kahn D, Ross R, Altshuler L, Cohen L.)
- At least 33% of women who have had postpartum depression have a recurrence of symptoms after a subsequent delivery (Epperson C N, *American Family Physician*, 1999)
- After the initial episode, women who have had PPD are at risk for both postpartum and non-postpartum relapses of depression. (Cooper and Murray 1997).
- *The course of PPD can be very changeable and inconsistent.* A woman might feel incapacitated by anxiety and hopelessness one day, and then feel relatively symptom free for some time, only to feel bad again with no apparent trigger or explanation.
- *The symptoms of PPD can be relieved and diminished within one to six months. But sometimes, depression can become chronic. Without effective treatment PPD may continue for as long as one to two years.* (O'Hara 1987) This is why it's so important to establish and maintain the most efficient and effective course of treatment and why we are developing that course of action in advance.

That's the not-so-good news. The good news is that with proper preparation and planning and a healthcare team that is mobilized on your behalf, we can intervene in ways that will minimize the likelihood that you will experience a depression to the same degree that you did previously. That's why we're doing the groundwork.

You will be prepared, you will be less anxious, and you will be in a better position to manage the outcome of this process.

Chances are good that you have been battling some of these thoughts about having another baby for a while now. Should we? Shouldn't we? If we should, then when? Should we wait until our child is older? Should we just jump in before we think about it too much and change our minds? What's the best timing?

Then, there's always the question of whether we should even consider another pregnancy at all. What about adoption? Or surrogacy? Or having an only child? Each of these options carries its own set of anxieties and rewards, and each entails a unique game plan. For our purpose here, we will gloss over these choices since our focus is on the experience of a subsequent pregnancy. Please understand that this in no way diminishes the relevance or magnitude of these choices for women who opt to consider them. If you are considering adoption or surrogacy, I would urge to you find support in your community so you can take advantage of all that is available to you.

◆

As we move forward in this process together, the following information will be most relevant to those of you who have, at least at this point, decided to proceed with the decision to try to get pregnant again despite the inevitable apprehension.

Undoubtedly, each woman has the potential to experience this process in a very unique way with a range of emotional responses. Still, we do find that there are patterns that develop which may help you understand where you are in terms this difficult decision. The following chart helps define the stages you might go through as you maneuver through this process. Keep in mind I have made the following assumption in this next section: If you are reading this, you are seriously considering getting pregnant, you have concerns about the outcome, specifically, how you will feel and function during the postpartum period, and these concerns are directly impacting your ability to be clear-minded and steadfast in this decision. Look at the following chart and see where you fit as the stages develop. You may find that you can relate to some of these stages, all of these stages, or none of them. Whatever the case, you can rest assured that you have a great deal of company in your quest for the picture perfect track. Sometimes, our hearts take over, and we proceed with great optimism. Other times, our brains win out and we start thinking of all the reasons we shouldn't do what we're doing and obstacles that can get in the way. Back and forth. Back and forth. All of a sudden, something that can feel so right at one moment can feel dangerously wrong. It's hard to know how to think it through. Or how to feel. The only sense you can make out of much of this is that it is not going to *make sense*. The best thing you can do is understand all of the factors involved in making this decision and equip yourself with the information and understanding that is necessary to guide you along.

STAGES	THOUGHTS AND FEELINGS	REASONING FEATURE	BEHAVIORS
I. INITIATION	"I want to have another baby" Hopefulness, cautious optimism, belief and trust in self, family.	Emotional, Affective	Dialogue with partner, gather information, explore options, asking opinions of others, fantasizing
II. REFLECTION	"I wonder if this is a good idea" Ambivalence, uncertainty, fearfulness, excitement, panic, disillusionment, inadequacy, self-doubt, guilt	Analytical	Revisit birth and postpartum experience, reassess trauma associated with experience, checking in on marriage
III. NEGOTIATION	"I think we can make this work" Curiosity, encouragement, confusion, enthusiasm, immobilization, emotional lability	Reconciliatory	Compromising, bargaining, challenging support resources, rapidly shifting moods and opinions
IV. RESOLUTION	"Everything will work out" Relief, lingering anxiety, reassurance, return to hopefulness	Rational	Increase the attractiveness of the chosen alternative "This is the best way to go because . . ."

The Initiation stage (What some women have referred to as the "What-am-I-thinking?!!" stage) is the first and earliest phase of the decision. It is typically characterized by more hopefulness and eager anticipation (this doesn't last long!) than anxiety and appears to be driven initially by the same blind faith that helps women forget how painful labor can be. It's the natural anesthesia that can follow an experience that may be painful and magnificently life-altering at the same time. It is during this time that couples begin to explore their options and confront early issues with wonder, questions, and possibilities.

For many (most) women with a history of PPD, this early stage is short-lived, primarily because the anxiety sets in almost immediately. As soon as the anxiety rears its ugly head, we are smack into stage two, which is the Reflection (or, the "Am-I-totally-nuts?!") stage. For what may be painfully obvious reasons, this second stage is the longest in terms of time, and the most difficult in terms of the emotional strain. Reflecting on the possibilities of what may or may not be generates considerable and constant anxiety. Are we doing the right thing? Could we be making a mistake? This is when the "what-ifs" start to intrude and may or may not continue throughout the process (and through pregnancy, childbirth and college!).

The reason this stage is most painful is because it causes you to think about all the things you have tried not to think about since your experience with PPD. The losses associated with PPD are immeasurable. Women have expressed this in many ways:

"I feel like I lost such valuable time with my baby."
"I feel like the first few months were a blur."
"I feel so guilty that I wasn't really there for my baby."

This is why so many women get stuck in stage two. While they're reflecting on their previous experiences, it can feel like the cost is too high. But the truth is, to move forward into the next stage of working this through, it becomes necessary to experience some of this ambivalence and yes, the anxieties as well, in order to sufficiently deal with and prepare for the issues facing you. This in turn will provide reassurance and information that is central to course of action you will take.

The third stage is the stage of Negotiation. At this point, although still confused about the right thing to do, couples often begin to see the light at the end of the tunnel. Seeking resources and information provides reassurance and early glimpses of cautious optimism replace some of the anxiety. Although there may continue to be a feeling of vulnerability and moodiness, most women begin to settle into thoughts of "maybe this will be okay after all." Hints of hopefulness combine with previous apprehensions to create a more positive vision of what may lie ahead.

Stage four is one of Resolution. Here's where we see the couple coming to terms with the decision to have another baby, but this is not to say that all their anxieties have left the scene. Although they may be diminished, anxieties will likely accompany the rest of the course of your decision making process, assuring that nothing is left to chance. This is because if any scenario can be imagined, from best to worst, it can be dealt with. *Resolution, here, refers to the determination to go forward, in spite of the anxieties.*

Along with other things that you might have learned serendipitously, your experience with PPD probably taught you that *you can function in spite of your anxieties and indeed, that you are able to function much better than you ever thought you could.* Getting rid of anxiety is not necessarily a primary goal. Functioning well despite the grip of anxiety or learning to coexist with it is by far the most productive and reassuring way to get on with your life.

Understanding PPD and
your risk factors

It all started in the summer. Katie brought her sweet Alison home in the sun-drenched August afternoon, after twelve hours of labor and the natural delivery she had so hoped for. The first few days were like heaven. Everything felt right.

But before long, Katie began to spend more and more time focusing on how her baby was doing and constantly questioning her own ability to make the right decisions. How much was enough, how much was too much—even a trip to the grocery store felt like more than she could handle. She was so tired, it hurt. Although her baby was managing to sleep several hours during the night, Katie found herself tossing and turning, with random thoughts racing through her head—what if the baby wakes up, what if I don't hear her, how am I going to be able to do what I need to do tomorrow if I don't get any sleep?

She remembers feeling so hot, the summer heat scorching her, burning from the inside out. She found it hard to catch her breath. Was it the heat?

Katie became increasingly sad and anxious and worried constantly about sweet Alison. She spent much of her day wondering how she would ever get anything done and after all, what was she thinking having a baby now when it was so hot and she was so tired. Maybe the fall would have been better? She knew how silly that sounded, but somehow, another time would have been better.

She would have been more prepared. She wouldn't be second guessing herself so much. Or would she?

Katie continued to worry. Was the baby warm enough, was she too hot, should she sleep on her side like that, would she die in her sleep, why was her breathing so shallow, why was she crying after she just ate, didn't she get enough food, did she get too much?

After a couple of months wondering and worrying, and her husband Mark encouraging her to get some support, Katie decided to call her doctor, who told her it was normal for her to feel weepy and unhappy for the first few months. At first she felt reassured by this, *see, it's normal. Everything is okay.* But after these feelings persisted for weeks on end, Katie knew this wasn't how she was supposed to feel. She knew something wasn't right. Although he did not say so outright, it was clear her doctor believed she was being overly dramatic. He recommended she see a psychiatrist. This confused Katie, she was almost relieved to hear that something might be wrong and she wasn't making this up, but somehow she felt her doctor didn't really take her seriously or understand what she was going through. She found it hard to follow through with his recommendations for fear that she would continue to be misunderstood.

The months passed and Katie struggled to keep up appearances as her efforts to remain grounded grew weaker. The anxiety settled in with a fierce grip and it became increasingly more difficult for her to differentiate what was "normal" and what wasn't. She began to isolate herself from her friends who seemed to be doing this mothering thing without skipping a beat. *Maybe this is just what being a mother feels like*, she thought. *Maybe it will never get better.*

Finally, when despair seemed her only alternative, she sought the advice of a close friend from whom she had tried her best to hide her symptoms. Immediately, she felt relief when her friend shared her own experience with similar feelings and gave her the phone number of a therapist who had helped her through it.

After one appointment with this therapist, Katie knew she was in the right place and felt comforted by the knowledge that she would not always have to feel this way. For the first time in a long time, she felt hopeful and encouraged about the days she had ahead of her. She understood she needed help to get better and felt relieved she didn't have to do this by herself any longer.

Postpartum depression is a mood disorder that can start anytime in the first few weeks after delivery or any time during the first postpartum year. It is a biological illness caused by changes in your brain chemistry. It is a medical condition that responds well to professional treatment, which is why women are encouraged to seek help as soon as they begin to question how they are feeling.

Sometimes women will tell me that they're not sure if they had PPD or not. This usually indicates that they experienced some degree of depressive symptoms that got better over time. Yes, that *can* happen but it's not recommended that you wait very long to see if these symptoms will disappear, since it's been proven that early intervention will speed recovery. Far too many women wait this out for too long, hoping their anxiety symptoms will "get better on their own," only to discover an increase in the severity of their symptoms, which ultimately makes recovery more difficult.

There are a number of reasons why the diagnosis of PPD can be difficult:

- *Misdiagnosis by medical professionals*: sometimes symptoms are misunderstood. For instance, since PPD can be an extremely agitated depression, sometimes a doctor will treat the anxiety and miss the underlying depression that may be at its core. Another reason is that symptoms of depression can overlap with what we believe is a "normal" part of new motherhood. Some examples of these would be fatigue, anxiety, feelings of inadequacy, crying. A doctor may interpret these symptoms as "normal" adjustments to motherhood or evidence of baby blues, even though in the case of a woman who's depressed, these symptoms may occur several months after delivery. Baby blues, the term which refers to these "normal" emotional and hormonal fluctuations (up to 80% of postpartum women experience this) is only applicable for the first two to three weeks postpartum. This is the time frame in which the hormonal influences of the delivery have the greatest impact. Any feelings of sadness, weepiness or anxiety, or other symptoms that linger beyond this time frame should be explored further for possible depression.

- *Mother's denial*: It is tempting to hope these painful feelings will just go away. This can be accompanied by an inability to acknowledge the pain or shame over the perceived "failure." It is often expressed by the woman in terms of her perceived emotional stability or ability to persevere in spite of the symptoms, "I can do this. If I just keep going, I'll feel better. Hopefully, this will go away or get better by itself. I just have to be strong."

- *Mother's inability to mobilize self*: The symptoms of depression can make you feel it is impossible to move in the right direction. As depression sets in with hopelessness, it can feel easier to stay put, remain inactive and apathetic.

- *Unsupportive spouse*: This may be a partner who doesn't take the symptoms seriously, or one who urges her to "snap out of it" or one who encourages her to "be strong" regardless of how bad she is feeling or how severe her symptoms are.

- *Desire for "quick fix"*: Most new mothers don't "have time" to be depressed. There is so much pressure to take care of so many things. Often, new moms put themselves at the bottom of their list of things to take care of.

- *Social/family pressures and expectations*: "This is supposed to be the best time of your life." Universally accepted and potentially harmful words. Need I say more?

Whether you had PPD that was diagnosed and treated by a professional or whether you experienced some vague symptoms that you now wonder how to classify, it's in your best interest to have a good understanding of what postpartum depression is because quite frankly, the risk for PPD is very high. *One out of every five women* will develop postpartum major depression.

Symptoms of PPD often include:

- A sad or depressed mood for much of the day
- Loss of interest in previously pleasurable activities
- Fatigue
- Guilt
- Difficulty concentrating
- Insomnia (sleep problems, difficulty falling asleep, or waking up after falling asleep and not being able to get back to sleep quickly, or waking too early)
- Appetite changes (either eating too much or not eating enough)
- Recurring thoughts of suicide
- Scary thoughts about harm coming to yourself or to your baby or loved ones
- Extreme anxiety
- Negative, intrusive thoughts
- Excessive worry
- Irritability
- Panic attacks (rapid breathing, feeling of impending doom)
- Feelings of inadequacy, low self-esteem
- Loss of motivation and withdrawal from others

As a rule, I trust a woman's instincts regarding her emotional state during the postpartum period. Women are typically quite in tune with their bodies and their own sense of well-being. At the risk of oversimplifying a complicated concept, I find that if a woman thinks there is something wrong, there usually is. That doesn't necessarily mean anything terrible is happening. But it does mean that things feel out of the norm and this needs to be addressed and taken seriously.

No doubt, at some point during the course of your illness and recovery, you asked yourself *why did this happen?* The hormonal changes of pregnancy and childbirth are known to contribute to a woman's risk for postpartum depression. In addition, caring for a newborn can be exhausting and overwhelming. Lack of sleep, unrealistic expectations, and social isolation can all play a role in the development of postpartum depression. This is why there is no single answer to the question of why this happened. Our best answer is that often, a number of factors combine and put a woman at risk for depression, some of which are hormonal, biologic, genetic, environmental, and psychological:

1) Some women may be more sensitive to hormonal changes, as is true with women who experience PMS.
2) Hormones, such as estrogen, progesterone, thyroid hormones, and cortisol may become unbalanced in women who are especially vulnerable.
3) Sleep deprivation or irregular, unpredictable sleep patterns will lower a woman's resistance.
4) If depression runs in your family, you are more at risk to experience it yourself. Understanding the course of any illness experienced by a family member may offer insight into the treatment of your own. In other words, if several family members have been successfully treated with a certain antidepressant, this would be useful information for your treating physician, because odds are that you will do well on the same antidepressant.
5) There does seem to be an association between the tendency to be a perfectionist or a "control freak" and difficulty in the postpartum period (when things are so drastically out of control for awhile!)
6) Pre-existing anxieties, predispositions to worry or ruminate, or obsessive qualities will put a woman at risk.
7) Any premorbid psychiatric history (that which occurred prior to PPD), such as obsessive-compulsive disorder (OCD), a previous episode of PPD, depression unrelated to childbirth, or

other diagnosed disorder for which you did or did not receive treatment will be risk factors for certain women.

8) History of early loss, trauma, abuse, or significant dysfunction in the family of origin will certainly affect a woman's ability to cope after the birth of her baby.

9) Other current outside stressors, such as major losses or changes related to: job, move, illness, death, divorce, for example.

Below is an expanded list of some of these and additional factors that may contribute to the emergence of depression after childbirth. Review the list to determine how many of these factors might have played a role in your previous depression. Next, see if any of these factors have changed since that time, either increasing or decreasing your risk. *Remember these factors do not cause depression, but they may increase your vulnerability to the recurrence of depression.* And also keep in mind that even if you do have a number of risk factors, this does not necessarily mean you will experience depression again. But it does mean you are armed with important information that may better protect you in the future.

- ❑ Previous personal history of postpartum depression, other clinical depression, anxiety or panic disorder, bipolar illness, eating disorders, or obsessive-compulsive disorder.
- ❑ A mother or sister who had PPD (genetic predisposition)
- ❑ History of severe PMS (hormonal vulnerability)
- ❑ Infertility treatment (although there is no documented relationship, the stress of infertility, hormonal treatments, and subsequent emotional upheaval can combine to create vulnerability.)
- ❑ Thyroid problems or family history of thyroid problems. (Fluctuating thyroid function after childbirth is common and can cause symptoms that mimic anxiety and depression.)
- ❑ Depression during pregnancy
- ❑ Unplanned or unwanted pregnancy
- ❑ Complicated pregnancy and/or delivery
- ❑ Extreme weight gain during pregnancy and/or difficulty losing weight after pregnancy

❑ Traumatic birth experience
❑ Chronic sleep deprivation
❑ Premature baby or other compromising conditions
❑ High-needs or colicky infant
❑ Infant with medical complications
❑ Difficulty or perceived difficulty with breastfeeding
❑ Abrupt discontinuation of breastfeeding
❑ Social isolation
❑ Marital instability
❑ Unsupportive partner
❑ Pre-existing and unresolved issues with partner
❑ Impaired family relationships, especially with your mother
❑ Lack of or distance from extended family
❑ Any recent adverse life event, such as difficulty at work, a recent move, a new job or other major change, the death of a loved one, financial problems
❑ History of childhood violence or abuse, emotional, physical, or sexual
❑ History of early major loss, especially a parent
❑ History of drug or alcohol abuse
❑ Extreme desire for control
❑ Birth control use (some association with worsening of depression for some women)
❑ Impaired self-esteem
❑ Tendency toward perfectionism

We know that risk factors do not *cause* postpartum depression. What risk factors do is set the stage for depression if the circumstances are right, making you more vulnerable to the illness. So it follows that even though we may not be able to actually *prevent* depression, it makes sense to take a look at areas in which you may not be as strong that may expose you to greater risk.

The list of risk factors above is extensive. Most of you will undoubtedly recognize many as playing a key role in your depression. Some are things you can do nothing about, they just are what they are. Others, you may want to take a closer look at to determine what you can do to better understand their impact and how you can react differently to preserve your highest levels of defense. Fortifying your resources will serve to protect you as well as reestablish a sense of control over future outcomes.

◆

Since we know that a history of PPD can make you susceptible to depression in general, not just during the postpartum period, it will be helpful to take a look at those areas of your life in which you feel fragile in some way. This fragility may be a result of lack of attention (an unrealized dream) or untouched status (a new unexplored idea) or abandonment (either by yourself or others who may reject or otherwise criticize) or a million other reasons that impact you and the things that are most important to you.

Start by making a list of the areas that you continue to feel need more attention. Do you still consider yourself vulnerable to depression (now) because of aspects of your life that remain unsupported? The term "unsupported" does not necessarily mean someone or something is not on your side. It means that there are areas which feel weak or that you feel are in conflict with your honest needs or desires. You may be ambivalent about or feel stuck by choices that you've made or paths you have taken. So the reference to feeling "unsupported" does not only refer to any lack of cooperation by others in your life who may express dissatisfaction in these areas. Rather, it refers to a more global sense of ambiguity or restlessness which you may hold deep in your spirit. The goal here is to help you identify and attend to those areas that may have been abandoned due to circumstances or merely by the tasks of daily living. Once looked at, these areas can be strengthened so that you can honor and embrace these parts of your true self.

Below, list the areas in your life which continue to feel problematic or create some conflict, either internal or with others in your life:

(Refer to the previous list of risk factors for direction. *Examples: career, stay-at-home status, marital relationship, body image, sexuality, isolation from friends, weight management, extended family, intimacy, to name a few*). It might help to think of starting each point with, "I wish I could . . ." or "If only . . ."

1)
2)
3)
4)
5)
6)

Next, circle one of the above items that makes you feel most at risk and write it again here, but this time, create a sentence out of it which states your concern *(ex: I think I would feel better if my husband agreed with my decision to stay at home and would stop pressuring me to go back to work)*: _____

_____

Are you able to put into words your concerns regarding these areas of vulnerability, and express them to those closest to you? If not, what seems to get in the way?

_____

Does it mean your partner is not on the same team? Does it mean you are getting pressure from other family members? Does it mean you are expressing yourself but no one is listening? Does it mean everyone is doing the right thing but you continue to feel misunderstood? Does it mean someone or something is sabotaging your efforts and desires? Does it mean YOU are getting in your own way? Does it mean you have not found the right avenue to express what you need? Does it mean you have not given yourself to permission to be honest about what you need or want?

Do your best to explore why you feel unsupported in these areas or why they continue to feel unfulfilled and try to put this into words. What is it about this situation or what is it about your personality or what is it about these specific issues in your life right now that make this an ongoing concern for you?

_____

_____

_____

_____

What, if anything, do you think YOU can do to start to make a difference in this area? In other words, let's assume you are the only one who has the power to strengthen these areas. It is not dependent on how others react to you (which may or may not be true!) It is important for you to focus on ways in which you can have an effect on changing things for yourself.

Pick one of your responses from the first numbered list above. It can be the same one you picked previously, or another one. Rewrite it below. Then write a couple of things you can do differently, perhaps an action taken, or a thought reframed or a behavior modified, that may create a shift in this area. Reframing your thoughts is one of the fundamental concepts of cognitive theory. This theory is founded on the assumption that we can learn to think differently and if we _think_ differently, we will _feel_ better. Consider this example of cognitive restructuring: "I failed this test because I'm a total loser. I suck at everything I do. I might as well not even try next time." We can reframe these statements into more positive thinking, such as "I didn't do as well on this test as I would have liked. Maybe I can do better next time. I'll contact my instructor and determine what steps need to be taken so I can improve." In this way, you can see how this process of thinking puts a new frame on a thought so it looks and feels different, even though it's the same picture.

Another example:

I feel guilty about going back to work and leaving my baby . . . *therefore I will:*

1) Explore options for working part time and spending more time at home with the children or find out about job sharing possibilities.
   OR
2) I will review with my partner how he feels about me staying home versus going to work.
   OR
3) I will look for a support group with other mothers who may be struggling with similar feelings
   OR
4) I will try to be kinder to myself and the choices I make and understand that the more I beat up on myself, the worse I will continue to feel.

Now let's try it out on one of your particular areas of concern:

One area of vulnerability from the above list I would like to work on right now is:

_____

Some specific things I can begin to do to help myself in this area so I feel less vulnerable are:

1) _____

2) _____

3) _____

4) _____

The work you have done here was not an easy task. You have been strong enough to dig deep inside a place you probably would rather not go. It's not easy to examine areas that need attention, especially if you think something about the way you deal with these issues continues to reinforce the problems. It takes great personal strength to put forth this amount of energy and to take responsibility for creating a new and different approach to getting the most meaningful and positive outcomes for overcoming your fears and working on areas you don't feel so strong in. Your commitment to continued recovery and optimal health is impressive and it will pay off in the end.

Taking a history

If you've been in therapy, you have probably spent considerable time looking at the impact of your depression and trying to make sense out of it all. It's quite possible that some of what transpired during your previous depression makes some sense to you now. For example, how your family history of depression most likely contributed to your experience. Or how your tendency to worry about details (which never caused a big problem for you before) developed into constant anxiety during the early postpartum months.

Though you have learned a great deal from your experience, about yourself, your marriage, your life, much of it still remains a mystery. That's because there aren't always clear answers to some of the questions that lurk ominously between what you've already been through and what you still face. Believe me when I tell you that I share your frustration. I would like nothing more than to say with absolute authority that I know exactly why this happened to you in the past and that we know exactly what to do to guarantee it will never darken your way again.

Regrettably, this is not so. The choice you can make, however, is to accept that sometimes you must move forward with the information you do have, in spite of what you do not know and cannot control, so you can improve the odds of a positive outcome.

One of the ways for you to harness this power over the ultimate outcome is to organize the details of your past history and treatment. This information, as well as the lessons you learned from the choices you made or those that were made on your behalf, will serve as a blueprint for your next pregnancy and postpartum experience.

It is well understood that depression can exhaust a woman's resources faster than almost anything else. Women who once felt competent and self-assured can lose confidence in their ability to make a decision. Women who once felt strong and capable can feel weak and defeated. Because of these symptoms, women are not always in a good position to advocate for themselves and the best healthcare while in the throes of depression. They may "know better" but the symptoms can interfere with their ability to intervene on their own behalf. Perhaps you heard your therapist say once or twice that you are much better at taking care of others than you are of yourself? This is because women who get depressed generally do not feel entitled to the care that they desperately need and in their effort not to impose what they perceive to be their burden onto others, they simply continue to make the needs of others more important than their own. Sound familiar?

Clearly, if you haven't learned this yet, learn it now. The *best* thing you can do for your self and for your baby and other children as well as your marriage, is to take care of YOU. If you do not learn how to make taking care of yourself a priority, the rest of our work here will be in vain. Taking care of yourself is not a luxury, it is essential.

A central part of taking care of yourself is making certain you are receiving the best possible treatment. Physicians and healthcare practitioners know a great deal and they are perhaps your greatest source of information and assistance. But they are not always right and they do not always have all the information you need. Therefore, one of the best ways for you to assure optimal care is to become informed so you can successfully advocate on behalf of your own healthcare. *You* are ultimately responsible for the care you receive and the choices that are made. Do not rely solely on the advice of others.

In this chapter we will take a close look at your previous treatment, what you have learned from this, and what you still need to know about the care you received and may receive in the future. Remember there are no absolutes about the treatment of depression. There is an abundance of literature supporting many different approaches. What works best for one person may not work well for someone else. Another unsettling reality is that if you ask ten experts what they would recommend for a course of treatment, you might get ten different responses. None would necessarily be the only "right" course. Nor would they all prove successful with every single individual. Even though there are tons of scientific theories and statistics that lead the way and influence the path of interventions for depression, much remains a matter of trial and error subject to individual differences and tolerances.

Therefore, the goal here is not to pass judgment on your previous course of treatment. Rather, it is to determine what worked best for you and what did not work for you, so you can make an informed evaluation of your treatment and create a plan that is customized to meet your particular needs. No one knows this information better than you do. You will be the manager of this project. And you will learn to let others know what you need.

Keep these points in mind regarding your healthcare professionals:

- If they aren't asking you the right questions . . . *you have to tell them, and if you can, tell them what the right questions are.*
- If they don't know how you are really feeling . . . *you have to express this.*
- If you feel they aren't taking you seriously . . . *you have to repeat yourself.*
- If you think you aren't being listened to . . . *you have to tell them this.*
- If you continue to think you aren't being listened to . . . *you have to consider finding another healthcare practitioner.*
- If you are afraid you are getting misinformation . . . *you need to challenge this.*

Far too often, depression during pregnancy and postpartum continues to be unrecognized and casually dismissed. Even though there is more understanding and awareness of these conditions than ever before, women need to be persistent in their quest for the best possible management of their healthcare. In addition, women seem to be busier and busier and families are often lacking the traditional comfort from their extended circle of relatives. As a result, you must take steps to become more and more accountable and to seek out, follow through, ask the right questions, and find the best answers.

To begin with, let's review your previous treatment.

One tool that has proven to be an effective way to process information and emotions is "journaling." Journaling is a personal form of self-expression that can actually help you communicate more efficiently with yourself. By writing down your thoughts and feelings, you can gain clarity and new levels of understanding. The journaling we will do here will be purposeful and focused on establishing a database from which to work later. All information you begin to record will become a critical part of your personal Postpartum Plan as you conclude this book.

Journaling your recent treatment history will help you run through some of the mechanics of how your illness was handled and provide the structure for lies ahead. It will also provide valuable and specific information for you to share with your healthcare practitioner.

Fill out the worksheet below as it applies to your most recent treatment for PPD. If you have experienced multiple episodes, either repeat it for each or extract the most relevant information from a previous experience and include it with your most recent.

Today's Date: _____

I am now _____ months / years postpartum

At the time I am writing this, I am, for the most part, feeling:

—	—	—	—	—	—	—	—	—	—	—
0	1	2	3	4	5	6	7	8	9	10

WORST I have ever felt   BEST I have ever felt

List the names of all the medications you took in the appropriate chart below.

(If you did not take medication, skip these questions) List either the generic or brand name, the therapeutic dose (what dose you ultimately achieved maximum results from, for example, if you were taking an antidepressant, started at 25mg for a week, increased to 50mg then gradually increased from 75 to 100mg and stayed at 100mg for the duration of your treatment, list 100mg), list any negative side effects from this medication, and rate how much these effects interfered with your normal functioning at the time. You may be able to get your prescription history printed out from your pharmacy.

- Medications I had the most success with:

Medication	Therapeutic dose	Side effects	Rate 0-5 5 being the most problematic

- Medications I did *not* do well on:

Medication	Therapeutic dose	Side effects	Rate 0-5 5 being the most problematic

- Medications (for depression/anxiety) I am *currently* taking:

Medication	Therapeutic dose	Side effects	Rate 0-5 5 being the most problematic

- How did you feel about taking medication *before* your experience with PPD?

_____

_____

_____

_____

- How do you now feel about taking medication *after* your experience?

  _____

  _____

  _____

  _____

- How do you feel, in general, about the possibility of taking medication again for a subsequent depression?

  _____

  _____

  _____

  _____

- If you had therapy, describe the course of therapy and how it was most helpful *(for example: how often did you meet, how long were you in therapy, how did you feel about your therapist?)*

  _____

  _____

  _____

  _____

- Complete this sentence: "I feel that the entire course of treatment (medication and/or therapy), for the most part, was . . ." _____

Why? _____

  _____

  _____

  _____

- Things that surprised or disappointed you about the course of treatment _____

  _____

  _____

  _____

- Further thoughts you have about the treatment you received

_____

_____

_____

_____

_____

- Is this (how you feel right now, at this point in time) where you expected to be, in terms of your recovery? If not, why not? And if so, how does that feel?

_____

_____

_____

_____

- What, specifically, about your treatment, had the most positive or negative impact on your experience with PPD?

_____

_____

_____

_____

- What, if anything, would you do differently next time?

_____

_____

_____

_____

- If you did *not* receive any treatment for PPD, would you do things differently, knowing what you know now?

_____

_____

_____

_____

- Do you feel your PPD has resolved? Why or why not? (*This question refers to the acute symptoms of PPD that brought you into treatment if you had it/or made you aware that you had PPD in the first place. It does not refer to longer term symptoms of anxiety or depression that you may continue to struggle with. This may be a difficult distinction to make but there is a difference. Resolution of your PPD may or may not mean the absence of ongoing, more chronic symptoms of anxiety or depression*)

  _____

  _____

  _____

  _____

- What do you consider to be your key issues that remain unresolved or symptoms that remain problematic?

1)

2)

3)

4)

5)

- List specific names of healthcare practitioners with whom you would like to share this information: (*Family doctor, OBGYN, therapist, psychiatrist, pediatrician*)

1)

2)

3)

4)

5)

6)

Assessing your resources

What got you through last time?
What should you have done differently?
What would make it better this time?
Who helped you most? How did they help?

Resources, in this context, refer to any available source of support that can be drawn upon as needed. In our first book, *This Isn't What I Expected*, Valerie Davis Raskin, MD and I separate this notion of support into two categories, *practical* support and *emotional* support. This distinction is important because there are times when a single person can provide a great deal of support of one kind but not another and knowing this ahead of time will lessen the likelihood that you'll be disappointed.

Practical support is anything someone can *do* for you. This may include help with the baby, the other children, the laundry, cooking, cleaning, babysitting, grocery shopping, and so forth. Emotional support is that which provides reassurance, guidance, validation, and comfort. This can be through words, or actions. It's something you might get automatically, or something you might have to ask for. The essential point is this: *You cannot expect people to know what you need unless you tell them.*

You cannot expect your support system to automatically be in place. You need to set it up. You need to reinforce it. You need to constantly reassess it and modify things if necessary. Most importantly, you need to convey what you need to the person or resource that is best equipped to make sure you get it.

Your list of support people and resources may include, among others:

- ❑ Partner
- ❑ Parents
- ❑ In-laws
- ❑ Siblings
- ❑ Partner's siblings
- ❑ Friends
- ❑ Neighbors
- ❑ Therapist
- ❑ Doctors and other healthcare practitioners
- ❑ Housecleaner
- ❑ Doula, baby nurse, nanny, baby sitters
- ❑ Church/synagogue
- ❑ Groups (support group, mother's groups, play groups)
- ❑ Structured settings with baby/children (ex: Gymboree, music groups)
- ❑ Structured settings without baby/children (ex: hobbies, classes)
- ❑ Gym or healthclub or other fitness outlet
- ❑ Other health programs such as hypnosis, yoga, acupuncture, chiropractor, massage, 12-step program, to name a few.

This list is not exhaustive, there are many more, to be sure. Do not underestimate the support that is available to you. The key is accessing it, communicating what you need, and making the most of what you have available.

Are these people or places you can count on? Are the people on this list aware of what you need from them? Do you need to sit down with any of them and discuss your concerns and your expectations?

Here are some additional points to consider regarding your resources and support network:

What will I do differently this next time?

1. _____
2. _____
3. _____
4. _____
5. _____

What will I try hard NOT to do this next time?

1. _____
2. _____
3. _____
4. _____
5. _____

What (or who) do I consider to be my greatest resource?

_____

What (or who) do I consider to be my most limited resource?

_____

What do I consider to be my strongest *personal* resource?

_____

What do I consider to be my weakest *personal* resource?

_____

The relationship you have with your partner is an essential piece to this puzzle and may, in fact, hold the key to how smooth your postpartum recovery is. As you already know, support can come in many forms and the support you get from your partner may be a bit tricky. Something that may appear to be or sound supportive may actually work against you. The definition of what is actually supportive for you is important for you to understand so you can sort out what's most helpful for you and what may get in your way.

Take, for example, some of the following statements:

- *"Honey, you're so strong. I know you can get through this."*
- *"Sweetheart, I agree with you, let's try to see if you can do this without medication. I bet you can."*
- *"If you run to your mother's every time you feel bad, you'll never learn how to take care of the baby."*
- *"You've been doing so well. You're crying much less now. I'm so proud of you. You're so strong."*
- *"Aren't you done with therapy yet? You look like you're doing fine."*

Any of these sound familiar? These are the words of very loving, supportive, thoughtful partners who are trying desperately to say the right thing and keep things on track. Can you see (or remember how it felt?) how these statements might unintentionally sabotage a woman's recovery efforts? There can be a hidden message in each of these examples that carries a heavy expectation that the woman either behave a certain way or feel a certain way, in order to uphold his belief in her resilience. Sometimes, this is due to his denial, sometimes it's due to his fear, sometimes, it's due to his desire for her to return to her "normal" self and previous level of functioning. In some cases, these mixed messages are a result of his impatience and frustration, but more often than not, it's the result of his anxiety and deep concern for his wife's well-being coupled with his very strong urge to say and do whatever he can to make it better.

None of this is intended to make either you or your partner feel critical of the support you are getting or giving. It is just a word of caution to alert you to the subtle impact that words can have and how carefully things need to be thought out and spoken in some circumstances.

Consider this scenario:

You're feeling depressed and paralyzed with panic. You've never felt so weak and tired in your life. You feel unable to get through the day without help and are afraid you will always feel this way. Your husband puts his arms around you and tells you how strong you are and how well he thinks you're doing. He possibly says this to bolster your self-esteem and help you see the positive in a negative situation. He's coaching you through the rough times and cheering you forward.

Instead of following his lead and thinking, *yes, he's right, I'm strong, I can do this,* you may only be able to hear that he has no idea how you're really feeling. *If you think I'm strong,* you think to yourself, *you either have no clue as to who I am, you're not listening to a word I've said, or you are totally in La-La Land.*

When we speak of support between a man and woman during a depressive crisis, we often have to cross gender boundaries, what *she* would want is not necessarily what *he* would want and so each is forced to identify with how and why the other is doing what he or she is doing. I know this can sound like a bunch of useless psychobabble, but it's significant because if left to its own devices, the instinct to support the other with familiar tactics may not only be ineffective, these strategies can potentially make things worse.

Imagine yourself in the bottom of an abyss. You're depressed. It's dark and deep. And there you sit. Your husband, who is worried sick about you, looks down into the dark hole into the void that surrounds you. He reaches in, stretching his long arms down to reach you. "C'mon," he urges "take my hand, I'll lead you back up." But you're so tired and weak. The thought of being lifted back to the real world feels like more than you can do right now. He continues to stretch his arm further to grab a bit of your self. You continue to sit motionless and sigh. What would feel better to you right now? Perhaps if he came down there with you, you could rest easy. Perhaps if he sat beside you with his strength and positive energy, you would find the force to move yourself closer to the opening. Perhaps if he didn't pull you up before you were ready, but acknowledged how deep and dark this was and could tolerate sitting there with you—that would help you feel understood and able to move. Perhaps.

The best thing for you to take away from this illustration is how important it is for you to express what you need and what you don't need to your husband. Otherwise, he's not going to know. This means be specific. Tell him that it makes you feel bad when he says a certain thing. Tell him how wonderful it sounds to hear him say such-and-such. Give him a script so he knows what to say and how to say it. This is something that is best to think about *now*, when you are not symptomatic and are able to think more clearly about what you may need in the future should symptoms arise.

◆

Be sure to check in with your partner at various times. Making sure the two of you know where the other stands is one of the most important things you can take care of right now. Chances are he's nervous about of all this too. And wants to proceed with the most cautious and practical means available. He may or may not feel he is ready to tackle what lies ahead. At this point, the best strategy for you to uphold is to facilitate an on-going dialogue. You might be wondering, why do *you* have to be responsible for this? You have to initiate this dialogue because frankly, you are probably better at doing this than he is. Be clear. Be honest. Be open to his concerns.

Make certain he knows:

- How you are really feeling.
- How he is really feeling.

- How worried you are and/or how excited you are.
- How important all of this is.
- How important it is for him to share his feelings with you.
- How important it is for you to share your feelings with him.
- What you are most afraid of.
- How he was most helpful or not helpful enough last time. (Be specific)
- How he can most help this time. (Be specific)
- Who your healthcare practitioners are and what their positions are regarding another baby.
- The risks involved in getting pregnant again.
- How essential it is that he remains connected to this process and to how you are feeling.
- How he is feeling as the process continues, how his feelings may change and how helpful it will be if he keeps you in the loop.

How have you changed?

I know that if I start this chapter by saying that some women have told me they think they are stronger and better women after their bout with PPD, I might lose a great number of readers at this very point. Declaring that depression can have a positive effect on someone's life may not be exactly what you want to hear. I dare say it comes perilously close to telling a woman with PPD that this is "the best time in your life." Not exactly what you want to hear, right?

Nevertheless, women *have* told me this and women continue to tell me that they have grown from their PPD experience. For some, their marriage got stronger as a result of learning how to communicate differently. For others, the increased self-awareness brought them to a new understanding of who they were and what they needed. Still others have confessed that the depression taught them how to take better care of themselves. These are just a few examples of how a disturbance as compelling as depression—that erupts at a time when families anticipate profound joy—can in the end bring forth new levels of understanding and compassion.

Janice was well into recovery from her PPD when she reflected on how her relationship with her husband had progressed.

It wasn't until after I was so much better that I was able to see how things had changed as a result of my depression. Barry and I had always taken certain things for granted and one of those things was that I would always be able to take care of everything. I wasn't ever good at asking for help, anyway. Well all that changed when I was sick. I waited and waited until things got so bad that I had no choice but to ask for help before I panicked myself to death. After eight years of marriage, I never knew how good it could feel to let my husband know that I needed him. And he tells me that it actually felt good for him to see me that way. Not that he wanted me to be sick. But it made him feel important and needed because I never expressed any of that before. It's much easier for each of us, now, to let the other know what we need.

Until now, we have focused more on the negatives PPD has created for you. Believe it or not, one of the more inspiring things you can do at this point in your preparation is to spend some time thinking about whatever positive role depression has played in your life.

- Are there ways in which you have changed since PPD that you think make you stronger or better?
- Have you learned things that came as a direct result of this trauma that may come in handy when you think about having another baby?
- Have you and your husband reached a different level of understanding since PPD?
- Are you better able to let go of things that you might have held on to longer before you had PPD?
- Do you notice that you are better able to let things stay out of place or not in perfect order or not as clean as you'd like without thinking your world will fall completely apart?
- Are you any better at giving yourself permission to slow down or take care of yourself?
- Do you recognize how important it is to ask for help when you're feeling overloaded or depleted?
- Do you now understand that taking care of yourself is not a luxury, but an essential part of being a good mother?
- Do you notice that you are much more aware of and sympathetic towards how others are feeling, particularly other new mothers who might be overwhelmed or depressed?
- Have you identified new sources of support? (the step-sister you never trusted who came through for you, the girlfriends from your PPD Internet message board)

- Do you find you are much better at intervening in order to take care of your emotional well-being when you feel particularly vulnerable?

These are some examples of how you might have changed. If any or many of these seem true to you, they mark valuable ways that you and/or your relationship have evolved toward a deeper and most likely, healthier state of being. That doesn't mean you enjoyed the process of getting there, by any means. But it does mean you can now appreciate some of the benefits you have worked so hard to achieve.

Section Three

MAKING THE DECISION

Anticipating medication questions

Pregnancy and breastfeeding

This chapter deserves an important disclaimer from the outset. First of all, I am not a doctor. The information in this chapter is not intended to serve as medical advice. *All* of your questions and concerns regarding medication must always be directed to your doctor. For that reason, I will not be discussing specific medications, side effects, why one is better than another, or what the current recommendations are. What follows instead is an overview of some of the most common concerns that women express regarding medication during pregnancy, postpartum, and breastfeeding and the very elaborate process of determining the optimal course to take. The purpose here is to offer general guidelines, rather than specific recommendations for your individual treatment plan.

By far the single most frequent question I get asked by a woman who has decided to proceed with another pregnancy after PPD is: What should I do about my medication? For women who have remained on medication since their previous PPD episode, the path to follow is not always a straightforward one.

- *Should I stay on my medication throughout the pregnancy?*
- *How do I know if the medication I am on is safe during pregnancy?*
- *Should I reduce the dose of my medication throughout the pregnancy?*

- *Should I taper down before I get pregnant and see how I do during the pregnancy?*
- *What if I stay on the medication and I still get depressed either during pregnancy or postpartum?*
- *Should I go off my medication and resume after the baby is born?*
- *Should I go off my medication and resume in the later stages of pregnancy?*
- *What if my symptoms get bad during pregnancy?*
- *What if I won't need the medication at all? Should I just wait and see?*
- *Will medication during pregnancy hurt the baby?*
- *If I go off and then need medication, do I take the same medication again that helped me last time?*
- *What if the medication doesn't help this next time?*

The decision to use antidepressants while pregnant or nursing is an extremely personal one. Your medical history and status are crucial factors in this equation. Another feature of this decision-making process is how you perceive your own risk taking behavior. One woman may say, "There is no way I'm going to take a pill while I'm pregnant, I would never do that to my baby. I'll just be depressed, that's okay." This woman believes that the risk of taking the medication is too great, while the risk of her depression impacting her baby is minimal. Another woman may say, "There is no way I'm going to let myself feel that way again. I'd much rather stay in control and take the medication while I'm pregnant so my baby will be protected." This woman, then, perceives the risk of *not* doing something, such as *not* taking the medication, as being the greater risk.

What is the "right" thing to do in each circumstance? It's so hard to know. Unfortunately, there's no easy or right answer that fits each and every woman. This is because each situation is unique and each woman responds differently to different medications and different doctors will recommend different options. Perhaps the biggest reason there is no good answer is the most disturbing of all, regardless of all the science and literature we have to substantiate our claims and recommendations, the ultimate outcome is still subject to unknown influences and a certain degree of chance. That's the part that doesn't feel good, I know. It would feel better if one could say with certainty, that *if you take such-and-such pill at this precise moment in time, it will directly impact the outcome in this known specific way.* Unfortunately, there is no such guarantee when we are dealing with intricate variables such as body chemistry, personalities, hormonal changes, environmental influences, and pharmacology. Not to mention, sleep deprivation! Therefore, as it becomes clearer just how many crucial components there are to making these decisions, it also becomes clear that your anxiety about this and preoccupation with making the best choice is quite reasonable.

Just to complicate things even further, the next thing to consider is who and how many people you discuss this with. There are so many options, so many opinions, and so much contradictory information. Here are some general tips to keep in mind:

1) *Be very wary of the Internet.* The Internet can be your friend or it can spin your head around with enough misinformation to propel your anxiety to previously unknown heights! If you tend to be a worrier by nature, you need to be particularly careful. You will find laypersons providing unsolicited medical advice and professionals endorsing a well-documented claim that is later refuted or disagreed with by another expert in the field. It can be a whirlwind of scientific data, personal opinions, impressive knowledge, scary misinformation, and inconsistent recommendations. So it bears repeating. Be careful. Be smart. And if you already know that you may have the tendency to over-react, obsess, or otherwise exaggerate the details of what you will be exposed to, do *not* go there.

2) *Don't ask too many people too many questions or you'll get too many opinions.* To illustrate, imagine taking a survey, asking

strangers on the street, for example, how they feel about an issue like breastfeeding. *Do you think a woman should breastfeed?*

- *Yes, definitely, it's the best thing for the baby.*
- *Yes, doctors recommend women breastfeed for the first year.*
- *Sure, I think doctors recommend women breastfeed as long as possible.*
- *Yes, don't doctors recommend women breastfeed until the baby weans himself?*
- *A woman should breastfeed only if she's stays at home full time. Not if she's working.*
- *Women can breastfeed when they go back to work. All they have to do is learn how to pump in between doing everything else.*
- *A woman should breastfeed if she has enough milk. I didn't have enough milk.*
- *Women should not breastfeed in public. Who wants to see that!*
- *Sure, women breastfeeding in public is a lovely display of honest affection and the maternal attachment.*
- *Definitely not. Women should not breastfeed, it's not natural.*
- *A woman should not breastfeed because it interferes with her ability to get a good night's sleep.*
- *Breastfeeding is far too demanding. It's hard enough being a new mother. She should have some time to herself!*
- *A woman should breastfeed only if she doesn't plan to supplement. Or the baby will get confused.*
- *A woman should breastfeed only if she supplements. Or she'll get too exhausted.*

That's fourteen different responses, some of which are rather contradictory, and I'm sure there are more! So it should be clear if you ask too many people the same question, you'll get too many answers and you'll end up more confused than when you started. The truth is, the issue of medication during pregnancy and lactation continues to be a point of research and debate, and if you asked a number of "experts" in the field, you would still get a number of different answers! That's why it's most valuable for you to follow the guidelines your doctor has set forth for you, assuming this relationship is one you have confidence in.

3) *Trust your instincts.* I know it's hard to know what the best thing to do is, when you're so overwhelmed with emotion as well as conflicting information. Try to think clearly. Try to think about what's best for you. This means what's best for your body, your spirit, your sense of well-being. Your comfort level is paramount. Coming to a decision that reinforces your anxiety will not help. Sit with yourself. Think about what you need and want to do. Make sure you are supported by your partner. Ultimately, you will be reassured along the way that you have made the right choices.

As a general rule, most experts try to avoid the use of medications during pregnancy and breastfeeding when at all possible. In fact, for women with more mild depressions where the symptoms do not significantly interfere with her functioning, choosing supportive psychotherapy over the use of medication is usually sufficient.

It's important to note that even with the most current literature to support the use of certain medications during these periods and more physicians being comfortable treating pregnant and nursing women with antidepressant medications, it remains a matter of significant ambiguity.

Studies do show that many antidepressants are "compatible" with breastfeeding. Keep in mind that all medications taken by the mother are secreted into the breastmilk. This amount will vary depending on the type and dose of the medication, how old the baby is, and the timing of the feeding, since the medications will peak at various intervals. To date, research results have not found exposure to most antidepressants to be associated with adverse events for the baby.

For obvious reasons, this issue of whether to breastfeed or not while taking medication remains quite controversial. While one woman is completely reassured by the available literature and comfortable with her decision to continue breastfeeding while taking an antidepressant, another one will be wary of this option and prefer to discontinue nursing when she starts the medication. If breastfeeding is important to you, let your doctor know the value this has for you. Also make sure you ask your doctor to clarify his/her position on this so you are one hundred percent sure you are in agreement.

Women suffering from depression during pregnancy or while they are breastfeeding are faced with the challenging option of whether to be treated with antidepressants during this time. The risks of treating with medication must always be weighed against the risk of no treatment. This risk-benefit analysis must always be very individualized, taking into consideration the severity of the illness, the stage of pregnancy or age of the baby, and mom's available support system. Ultimately, the goal is for a healthy mother and a healthy baby.

Key research conclusions:

- Whenever possible, women should be encouraged to engage in psychotherapy or supportive counseling unless moderate to severe symptoms warrant medication use.
- Postpartum depression has been shown to have a negative effect on parenting and attachment as well as infant development (Cooper P, Murray L 1996)
- Many medications for the treatment of depression have been studied and are considered compatible with pregnancy and breastfeeding. (Spencer, J 2001)
- All antidepressants are excreted into breastmilk to some degree. (Wisner KL 2002)
- A mother who is pregnant or who's breastfeeding should be treated with the lowest effective dose in order to minimize fetal or infant exposure to antidepressants.
- Medications that are safe during pregnancy are not always safe in breastfeeding mothers. (Spencer, J, 2001)

- Studies demonstrate no adverse effects of antidepressants when minor traces are detected in the infants' blood. (Stowe ZN et all, 1997)

♦

No doubt, you have already experienced some degree of this uncertainty in relation to your previous experience with PPD or just with becoming a mother; how to do what, when to do it, why, and so forth. There will always be loving, well-intentioned friends, family members, neighbors, strangers, as well as your healthcare professionals, eager to share their views on which road you should take. Sometimes it will be because you asked for their opinion. Sometimes it will not.

But the upshot is this: When it comes to making a decision as important as how to proceed with your medication, you cannot afford to wrestle with misinformation and doubtful opinions. So decide right now who you will discuss this with and on what you will base your decision. More often than not, this will mean an open dialogue between you and your partner. Next, I would advise you have a consultation with your prescribing physician (psychiatrist, OBGYN, family doctor) and your therapist if you are seeing someone. I would leave it at that.

These discussions with your healthcare providers will not just be a one time event. It may be a process whereby you review what your experience was, what your expectations are, what you are afraid of, what is primarily influencing your preference right now, and how their expertise can best guide your through this process. Some important points to go over with your healthcare professional (these are in addition to the medication review worksheets you have already completed):

1) Discuss why you are in favor or opposed to staying on or taking medication during pregnancy or the postpartum period.

2) Discuss openly what concerns you the most about medication.
3) Ask your healthcare practitioners about their specific experience and expertise using meds during pregnancy/postpartum/breastfeeding if applicable, and what their comfort level is.
4) Make sure your partner is an active part of these dialogues, either physically present at the consultations, or in direct conversation with you regarding the specifics.
5) Make certain your partner feels free to express whatever concerns, hesitations, and disagreements he may have to insure you both are on the same page.

Tips for you and your doctor to keep in mind if you plan to breastfeed and take medication:

- Talk to your doctor about taking a medication with a shorter half-life. This means it will be easier for your baby to metabolize, resulting in less risk of the drug accumulating in his system.
- If you need to take a medication that causes particular concern for you, you should talk to your doctor about taking it right after feeding your baby. Since most medications reach peak concentration a few hours after taking them, this will give the medications time to clear your system before the next feeding time. Perhaps your pharmacist can also offer assistance with this.
- If you take a medication that requires one single dose a day, it is recommended that you take it just before the longest sleep interval for your baby. This is usually right after the last feeding before putting your baby to sleep for the night.
- If you need to take a medication that requires multiple dosing, it is recommended that you nurse your baby immediately before you take your medication dose.

(Hale, T., 1998-99. and Lawrence, R., 1999.)

A final word of caution:

One of my deepest concerns rests with women who are determined to continue breastfeeding at all costs, who are resistant to taking medication, and who continue to struggle with severe symptoms that would respond well to medication. I worry about these women because I understand how difficult is can be to think clearly when depressive symptoms impair judgment. I understand how easily a mother may suspend her own well-being on behalf of what *she thinks* is best for her baby. I also understand how dangerous this preference to continue to breastfeed and not take medication can potentially be. The trade-off for this choice, at its most extreme, can be disastrous.

If your symptoms are significant enough that medication is necessary, the risk of not taking the medication can be extremely high. Symptoms such as distorted thinking, marked inability to function (including disturbances in sleep, appetite, and concentration), impaired attachment to your baby, obsessive or negative intrusive thoughts or images, and suicidal thoughts are just some of the symptoms that indicate the need for medication. *Not taking the medication is not an option.*

Therefore, the bottom line is this: If you are suffering from a severe depression and have been told by your doctor that you need medication and you are breastfeeding—you have two choices:

You can continue to breastfeed and take the medication,

OR

You can stop breastfeeding and take the medication.

Those are the choices you have.

In summary, although we know that the use of antidepressant medications during pregnancy and breastfeeding carries some potential risks, it is often the case that the benefits of treating maternal depression and maintaining breastfeeding seem to outweigh the risks of exposing your baby to small amounts of the medication. Unquestionably, this decision should always be individualized, balancing your needs, desires, and expectations with your symptoms and recommendations for treatment.

Medication before PPD occurs?

For women with a significant history of depression, and in particular, a history of a previous postpartum depression, the use of preventive (prophylactic) antidepressants may be warranted during pregnancy and the postpartum period. Although I cannot overemphasize the importance and value of psychoeducation as an integral part of the preparation, sometimes it's simply not enough. If you, your partner, and your doctor determine that starting medication in late pregnancy or the early postpartum period is reasonable, most agree that your doctor should prescribe the antidepressant that has worked for you in the past and certainly avoid those that have not. When antidepressant medication is initiated late in pregnancy as preventative treatment, it is typically initiated some time in the last month before delivery. The specifics of this intervention will vary greatly with each prescribing physician, so make sure you familiarize yourself with your doctor's preference and past experiences of success.

The research we have on the use of postpartum prophylactic therapy is limited. Yet, clinicians agree that their own clinical experience has shown that these early interventions do tend to work at reducing the likelihood of PPD recurring or reducing the impact of the illness if it does recur. This seems to be particularly true for women who experience symptoms of depression during pregnancy or who experience a high degree of stress during the postpartum period.

Ultimately, if we are talking about taking medications during pregnancy or while breastfeeding, or whether we are deciding to start medications at the end of pregnancy or right after delivery, or if you are wondering whether you should stop breastfeeding or not, only one thing is clear. There is no perfect decision, and no decision is without risk. Keep an open mind, keep an open dialogue and above all, be true to what's most important to you, while carefully considering the advice of your treating physician. Make a plan that is acceptable to your doctor, your partner and yourself. Then, make an alternative plan you can use as a backup.

The wisdom of your decision

Given that there are no perfect decisions and since each decision you make along the way has its own associated risks, it would follow that you should expect some anxiety to accompany you during this journey. It would be nice if we could, through the wisdom of our quest for expert knowledge and guidance, experience total peace and harmony along the way. It's frustrating not to know what's ahead of us or how things are going to turn out. Try as we might to control the uncontrollable, ultimately life teaches us that there is little we can do to avoid uncertainties.

Most likely, you are someone who identifies strongly with the need to be in control. Everyone likes to be in control. Still, some of us work harder at maintaining our hold on things, partly because it feels better to be in control and partly because the prospect of losing that control feels unbearable. Each of these is misleading, however. Holding on to something because you're afraid to let go creates a false sense of security, an illusion of control. Letting go, on the other hand, can lead to promising results. For instance, imagine holding a filled water balloon in the palm of your hand. It starts wobbling around and soon it's hard to keep balanced in your open hand. Fear of dropping it and splattering it all over, your instinct may be to clutch it tightly to hold it in place and keep it from slipping. But what happens if you do that? Most likely, the pressure from the water balloon will resist your grip and it will either bounce out of your hand onto the ground or burst open squirting water all over the place. This teaches us that squeezing tightly is not the best way to gain control over an unsteady water balloon. The best way to hold on and maintain control is to let go, to release the grip, to open your fingers out and let the balloon find its natural resting spot. In the same way, by letting go, not by holding on or by gripping tightly, we can keep our equilibrium and as a result, maintain a good deal of control.

Here are some examples of things you may do that may inadvertently sabotage your efforts at maintaining control: (Some of these tendencies are okay to an extent; It's when they become excessive that they become counterproductive. Sometimes, that's a fine line to distinguish!)

1) Ask lots of questions or lots of people's opinions or search relentlessly for information. *(Which medication did YOU take, did you breastfeed, did your doctor say that was okay? I read that one wasn't good for breastfeeding.)*

2) Remain doubtful of your position or decision and constantly seek reassurance and validation *(Do you agree with me or think I'm doing the right thing?).*

3) Ruminate or obsess about the available choices or choices already made *(maybe if I think about this long enough and hard enough, I'll convince myself that I've chosen the right way and am doing the right thing).*

We yearn for predictability. For example:

• If I take this medication, can you guarantee I won't get depressed?
• If I breastfeed while taking this medication, are you positive my baby won't be affected?
• If I decide not to take medication, do you promise I can take it later and it will still help?
• If I do get depressed again and I go to therapy and do what I'm supposed to do, will it be as bad as last time?
• If I tell my husband exactly what I need from him, will this ensure that he'll be able to support me better than last time?
• If I decide not to have another baby, are you sure I will regret it?
• If I decide to adopt, does this mean I'll never get depressed again?

So much of this entire process would be easier if we just had some kind of warranty to secure the desired outcome. If you do such-and-such, this will definitely happen. The security of a known structure that provides predictability makes us feel safe and comfortable. The unknown is what makes us afraid.

The best we can do with this concept of the unknown is to accept it. Accepting that some things will remain out of your control regardless of what you do and how you prepare will help you ride out the course with the least amount of discomfort, no matter which way it takes you. The picture looks like this: you strategize, you anticipate, you do your research, and you set things in motion in order to prepare for this next phase of your life. Simultaneously, you recognize that despite this hard work you are doing, there will continue to be parts of your life that remain out of your control. Embracing this apparent contradiction will help you balance your expectations with the reality that life brings to you. In this way, you will feel more balanced as you move forward.

Here are some things that you CAN do to increase your feelings of control while you face such an unpredictable course of events:

1) Trust your instincts.
2) Trust your doctor and other healthcare practitioners.
3) Expect and allow the presence of anxiety and do not misinterpret that anxiety as evidence that you are doing the wrong thing.
4) Give yourself permission to experience this anxiety along with the confidence that you have made good decisions.
5) Do your best not to second guess yourself. After such a comprehensive and thoughtful process, give yourself the benefit of the doubt. Believe in yourself and your choices.
6) If you are in need of reassurance, find one or two people you trust and direct your questions and concerns only to them. Avoid the temptation to ask too many people or seek too much

information, hunting for the perfect response. This will only confuse you.

7) Try to tolerate the uneasiness this decision-making process may produce. Some of it is par for the course. Don't beat yourself up. Expect this process to be difficult. Don't expect this to be any easier than it is.

8) If you are leaning toward a decision that brings significant pain or loss, such as a decision not to have another baby or the decision not to breastfeed—do not forget to pay special attention to how this may affect your spirit and your body. Bear in mind that just because you are feeling pain associated with a decision that brings loss, this does not mean you've made the wrong decision. It means there is a loss involved and grief is a natural response to this loss. Nurture yourself and spend time soothing your soul with things and people and places that feel especially good to you.

Section Four

PREPARING FOR PREGNANCY
AND ANOTHER BABY

Fortifying your resources

Pregnancy as preparation

One of the best things you can do to prepare for your next postpartum period is to use your pregnancy as an operational foundation. Your pregnancy will serve as a command center, creating the time-frame and structure you and your partner need to set in motion the planning that may, up until this point, have been speculative. Things need to be settled upon and finalized now. Decisions need to be made. Your pregnancy is the optimal time for you and your husband to prime yourselves for all you have anticipated and all that is left to be planned. Whether you are feeling good physically and emotionally during your pregnancy, or whether you are feeling symptomatic and in treatment, your partner needs to be completely engaged in this process at this point.

If you are currently pregnant, it's likely that you're feeling anxious, eager, excited, nervous, and maybe even wonderful. There is no time like the present to focus on what needs to be reviewed and what details still need to be arranged to move this process along. Nothing will help you feel more in control right now than improvising a recipe that can carry you through the first few weeks postpartum, ensuring that everything you can possibly foresee has been taken into account.

When Jessie was seven months pregnant, she told me about her worry that she wouldn't always feel as good as she feels now and "what if" she sinks rapidly despite her best preparations? "It's as if right now, I know, but I might not, later. Like, I know what signs to look out for but I'm afraid if I'm in the middle of it, I won't be able to see it." Jessie was right about part of her worry. Sometimes, in the fog of depressive thinking, we might not see what we think we *should* be able to see when we are thinking clearly. In other words, if you're thinking now that lack of sleep and irritability will increase your risk of depression, after four straight nights of sleeplessness and unrelenting fatigue and irritability, you may resist the notion that these may be warning signs and continue to keep on doing things that are not in your best interests despite words of caution from others. This is because people don't think clearly when symptoms of depression set in. So Jessie has a good point. How can she "warn" herself *before* she feels this way that she might feel this way?

She decided it would be helpful to write herself a note, a script of sorts. As if her depressed self was separate, somehow, and might need the wisdom that only her current healthy voice could articulate. Below is what she came up with. You might find it helpful to modify this to fit your particular symptoms or areas of vulnerability.

"Talking Points" are lists that Jessie came up with that she kept close in view for easy reference during her postpartum recovery. It served as a reality check and a gentle reminder of what she needed to know. Review her lists. Check the statements that apply to you and add any additional points that are relevant to your personal experience. Remember, *these are lists that applied to one particular woman*, although I am certain many women can relate to most of them. Be sure to add your own contribution and cross off the ones that do not apply so the lists can be customized to best meet your needs. This will also be reviewed and consolidated in the chapter to follow where we create your personalized postpartum plan.

List of my warning signs

- Can't make a decision
- Can't feel comfortable with anything
- Nothing feels right or good enough
- Obsessing over little things or everything
- If I feel: "like I'm having an out of body experience, like I want to crawl out of my skin, or every time the baby cries I want to jump out the window"
- If a change in the routine bothers me
- Too tired, too irritable, too angry, too anxious
- All I want to do is sleep
- If I feel like I can't take one more minute
- _____
- _____
- _____
- _____
- _____

List of comforting words

- This feeling (that I want to jump out of my skin), or any feeling that feels so awful will get better. I won't always feel this way.
- If I feel confused, it's okay. I can ask someone to help me.
- If I don't feel as good as I think I should, that doesn't mean anything terrible is happening. But it does mean I should check it out.
- I can (and should) tell my husband and therapist/doctor how I'm feeling.
- If there is noise or racing thoughts in my head, someone else needs to know.
- If I don't feel close to my baby right away, that's okay. I know I will eventually bond in a meaningful way. It's all right to have whatever feelings I have or I don't have and I don't have to feel any particular way at the beginning.

- If I have bad thoughts, I have to remember that these are symptoms and I don't need to be ashamed or secretive about them. I can (and should) tell someone I trust.
- Everything I am feeling that is scaring me or making me feel bad is a symptom. It is not about who I am or what kind of mother I am.
- _____
- _____
- _____
- _____
- _____

What helps me

- I need to make sure I get enough sleep
  —someone sleeping over, me sleeping out
  —ear plugs
  —room darkening
  —sound machine (white noise)
- Help in the house
  —Nanny, housekeeper, babysitter, doula, nurse, relative
- Remove all dangerous substances from the house (It's awful to see this in print, but many women tell me it feels better to know that all temptations are removed from the house. Any sleeping pill, even Tylenol PM, can have frightening power when you are willing to do anything just to sleep. Guns should not be in the house. It is the best time to make decisions about whether sleeping pills and potentially addictive medications, such as anti-anxiety medications, should be kept by the husband. And these difficult but crucial decisions should be discussed at this time, before possible volatile situations are encountered.)
- _____
- _____
- _____
- _____
- _____

To my husband: here's what I need to hear you to say

(These things are hard to believe when you're feeling depressed, but very important for your husband to continue to say them to you)

- I'm not going anywhere. I will not leave you. No matter how bad you feel or how long this takes.
- Go lie down and try to feel better, rest. I'll take the baby.
- I know you won't believe me when I tell you, but you will feel better again. I've seen you feel this bad and I've seen you get better. I know this to be true.
- Tell me what you want me to do to help. Would it help you if I..........?
- _____
- _____
- _____
- _____

Specific things we need to do *differently* this time

- Put the baby in the crib, not in our room.
- Don't wait so long before asking my mother to come help.
- Have the sitter come at least once a week whether we have something planned or not.
- Check in with each other at least once a day to see how we are doing and what we need.
- Do not assume that everything is okay with the other partner unless we check it out.
- _____
- _____
- _____
- _____
- _____

If you are depressed during pregnancy

Despite the fantasy and expectation that pregnant women glow with eager anticipation of the upcoming exquisite event, a significant percentage of women suffer from symptoms of depression during this time. Recurrence of depression during pregnancy is a significant issue that deserves attention. Research now suggests that women who have a history of depression at any time in their lives are twice as likely as other women to experience depression during pregnancy. One of the reasons that depression during pregnancy (antepartum or prenatal depression) goes unrecognized is because many of the symptoms we associate with depression are also common with any pregnancy, such as fatigue, insomnia, and mood changes. This can make it difficult for both the woman as well as her physician to detect the onset of depression.

Symptoms of depression during pregnancy are similar to symptoms of postpartum depression.

Some common symptoms of depression during pregnancy:
- Sleep disturbances
- Excessive anxiety and ruminations
- Preoccupation with baby's health
- Extreme fatigue
- Feelings of sadness, hopelessness
- Feelings of guilt
- Difficulty concentrating
- Negative, intrusive thoughts
- Uncertainty about the decision that has already been made to go ahead and have the baby
- Panic or irrational feelings of terror or dread
- Thoughts that baby would be better off without you

What you need to know:

- Contrary to what may be a popular belief, pregnancy does not protect a woman from depression.
- Approximately 10-15% of pregnant women experience symptoms of depression, which are similar to symptoms of depression at other times but may focus more specifically on the pregnancy itself and/or the health of the baby.
- Women who have had major depression in the past are at greater risk for depression during pregnancy.
- If you experienced a depression during a previous pregnancy, you are definitely at an increased risk for depressive symptoms with a subsequent pregnancy.
- Women with histories of mood or anxiety disorders who decide to stop taking their medications during pregnancy are particularly vulnerable to depression.
- There is much data to suggest that certain medications may be used during pregnancy without significant risk to the fetus.
- If you experience a depression during pregnancy, you are at an increased risk for postpartum depression.
- Many medications are considered acceptable for treating depressive symptoms during pregnancy but the risks must always be weighed against the benefits on an individual basis.

One of the most vital tasks at hand is to educate everyone who may be affected by this situation about the very real risk of depression during a time most people do not expect such a disturbance to occur. Pregnancy can make women vulnerable to emotional swings caused by hormonal and physical changes, as well as psychological ones. The challenge here is to determine with the help of your doctor what is within "normal limits" and what needs closer attention.

If you think you might be experiencing symptoms of depression during your pregnancy, it is vital that you receive prompt treatment so that symptoms do not continue or worsen.

The risks of not treating depression during pregnancy can be significant. Untreated depression during pregnancy can:

1) Interfere with your ability to enjoy the pregnancy
2) Prevent you from taking good care of yourself, including prenatal care
3) Impair nutrition, sleep, and your ability to follow medical recommendations
4) Impact some women's ability to form a healthy attachment to the baby
5) Increase the tendency to drink or smoke
6) Be linked with prolonged or premature labor or low birth weight
7) Increase your risk of postpartum depression

The impact on your family

Your marriage

If you have struggled with depression after the birth of a baby, you know only too well why we say that postpartum depression is an illness that affects the entire family. In fact, one of the features that sets PPD apart from "regular" depression (one that is not related to childbirth) is the urgent demand of a newborn claiming priority. A screaming baby is unmindful of his mother's weary indifference or paralyzing anxiety. The real agony of this paradox is that depression itself is an incredibly self-absorbing condition. By definition and at its very core, it is an illness that forces a woman to remain relentlessly locked within herself, what one woman called, "the curse of self-awareness": *am I good enough, am I doing this right, will I ever be able to do this, will I ever look good again, will I ever feel like myself again, why is everyone else doing it so easily and so well, can they tell how hard this is for me, can they tell how bad I am at this, will I ever love this baby, will my husband leave me?*

When Anne was four months postpartum, she told me she wanted to bring her husband in to the next session. I encouraged her to do that and asked why she was asking for this at this time: "Keith is such an awesome guy. He's put up with so much. He's been there for me since the baby was born, you know that. He comes home from work, throws a load of laundry in, takes the baby and carries him around the house while he straightens up the mess I've left in every corner. He never complains about it and never asks when I'll be done with all this stupid depression stuff." The tears spill down her cheeks as she continues to talk about Keith, "I mean, how much of this can he take? When will he decide enough is enough? I'm so afraid one day he will just decide not to come home again. I know I wouldn't blame him if he did that."

Anne and Keith had a very strong relationship. They had been married for four years before their baby was born and had endured an earlier episode with depression early in their marriage. Keith had no intention of ever going anywhere and was incredibly committed to the marriage and to supporting his wife. He was, as Anne noted, extremely supportive and very good at doing exactly what he needed to do during the crisis. Her fear of his leaving and her guilt over the burden the illness imposed upon him were pervasive. The more supportive he was, the guiltier she felt.

Everyone agrees that the impact PPD has on the family is significant and undeniable. In view of that, the sensible direction to take is to understand how *your* family did (previously) and how it will (the next time) respond to the challenge of PPD. This next section focuses on the relationship with your husband and it would be most helpful if you review these questions and answers with him. Establishing an open dialogue about both the positive and negative aspects depression can have on the marriage is essential to smooth postpartum recovery. It is not enough to pretend everything was okay. It will not be helpful to assume he knows what he should or should not do. It should not be acceptable to you that even though he reassures you that everything will be okay, he does not take the time to actually sit down with you for as long as it takes and to get busy doing this work right now.

Men don't have it easy in this scenario, for sure. Just ask any husband of a woman with PPD, it's like walking on eggshells. In my book, "The Postpartum Husband," I point out how difficult it can be for men to "say the right thing" when their wives are suffering from depression:

♦ If you tell her you love her, *she won't believe you.*
♦ If you tell her she's a good mother, *she'll think you're just saying that to make her feel better.*
♦ If you tell her she's beautiful, *she'll assume you're lying.*
♦ If you tell her not to worry about anything, *she'll think you have no idea how bad she feels.*
♦ If you tell her you'll come home early to help her, *she'll feel guilty.*
♦ If you tell her you have to work late, *she'll think you don't care.*

Sometimes, it can feel like a lose-lose proposition. Furthermore, husbands who try desperately to say or do the right thing can wind up innocently aggravating the situation.

For instance, here are some subtle ways your devoted and well-meaning husband can make you feel worse without knowing it:

• *Expecting you to "be strong."* Whether he expresses this in words or not, this expectation can pressure you and make it difficult for you to let him know how bad you are truly feeling. A reference to your strength at a time when you feel incapacitated by weakness can be interpreted by you as his denial or lack of connection to how you are really feeling.

• *Telling you how well you are doing before you think you are.* He may actually be right about how well you are doing, but if he says it before you are ready to hear it, you may resist hearing it or think he doesn't understand, which isn't necessarily so. What helps is for him to be specific about how he thinks you are doing better and most importantly, preface his statement with a disclaimer such as "I know you're not quite back to your old self, but I notice it's getting easier for you to . . ."

• *Asking you if you're almost done with therapy or making a comment about how much it costs.* He means well, but he probably has no idea how that can instantly get you off track. What he thinks is a reasonable and perfectly appropriate concern can in truth, defeat the process. His attempt to be practical can be misperceived by you as criticism or it may make you feel full of shame and unworthy of the expense and burden.

• *Asking, hoping, expecting, desiring, demanding, requiring, or pleading for sex.* Most postpartum women (whether they are depressed or not) find they are not ready to have sex quite as soon as their husbands are. Of course, this is a generalization and many women are eager to resume their sexual relationship, but wanting sex soon after the birth of a baby is the exception. When you add depression to that picture, sex becomes just one more thing a woman feels she cannot do. She's too tired, she's too fat, she's too anxious, she's too preoccupied, she's too restless or scared. Whatever her reason, whatever her symptoms, sex is rarely on the top of her list of things to take care of. Her husband, however, may think this would be a nice, gentle, loving way to express how much he loves her and surely, it will help her feel better. *Wrong.* Instead, what she might prefer is to be held, snuggled, hugged, touched, spoken to, or caressed. Or she might want to be left alone. Or she might not be sure. This needs to be checked out, by asking by talking, by sharing. If sex becomes part of this picture, that's great. If not, it needs to wait.

Think about the unfinished task of letting your husband know what he did last time that worked or didn't work. This is crucial. If you've gone over this together before, that's good, you'll go over it again now and you'll feel more confident about it. If you haven't yet gone over this, you should, otherwise you run the risk of 1) harboring resentment over losses from previous experience 2) staying or getting angry and his failure to meet your needs and 3) experiencing a repeat performance of everything you didn't like last time.

The following is a two-part exercise. The first part is completing the sentences. The second part is having a conversation with your husband about it.

When I had PPD the last time:

1) It felt so good when you _____
2) I never told you how much _____
3) Sometimes, it made me feel bad when you _____
4) I know you were trying to help, but it was hard for me when you _____
5) One of the things I needed most from you was _____
6) Thank you for _____
7) When you get tired or frustrated or angry, I hope you can _____ _____
8) I know now that sometimes_____
9) Sometimes I secretly wished _____
10) I believe that the two of us _____

Remember, your husband will not know how you feel or what you are thinking unless you tell him. Even if you have talked about these matters before, they bear repeating. You are the one in the best position to let him know how he can best meet your needs. He can try to remember, he can try to read your mind, he can make it up as he goes along, or you can just tell him again. You can resent him for making you reiterate what you need, you can wait and see if he figures it out on own, you can wonder if he ever listens to you, or you can just tell him again.

Your children

Of great concern to many women is this burning question, "How will I be able to take care of my toddler if I get depressed again?" This brings to light two points, 1) how does maternal depression affect the toddler and 2) what can you do to best protect this child and minimize any negative consequences from the depression.

There is evidence that suggests maternal depression can certainly have negative effects on children, depending on the severity and chronicity of the illness. The good news is that depression responds well to treatment. As noted previously, the absolute best defense against depression and its potentially detrimental effects is *early identification and intervention.*

Because depression can be such a self-absorbing illness, some women worry that they will be too preoccupied with their own mental health or distracted by their symptoms to adequately care for their children. Sometimes, this is the case. More often than not, however, women find the resources they need to either augment their care or temporarily substitute for it, providing ample support and back up as needed. During a PPD crisis, the most important thing for your children, whether it's your newborn or your toddler, is that they receive consistent loving attention from a devoted caretaker. In an ideal world, this would come from the children's parents. When circumstances prevent that in the short term, alternate caretakers can fill in, preferably with the children's father in the front line.

Here are some points to keep in mind to manage PPD with respect to your children:

1) During depression, you *may* be less responsive, less interested, or less able to meet the needs of your children. *Do not hesitate to let others help you.*

2) During depression, you *may* feel more critical, more negative, and more insecure about your mothering skills, your ability to bond or your relationships with your children. *Do not judge yourself too harshly during this difficult time.*

3) Studies have shown that when mothers who are more sensitive by nature are able to be aware of their children's needs in spite of their own depressions, the impact on the children is less apparent. (Edhborg M, Seimyr, L, Lundh, W, & Widstroem, A, 2000). Being sensitive to the particular needs of each individual child, to the extent possible within the limitations of the illness, is beneficial. *Do not relinquish your innate*

*sensitivities and sensibilities to the wrath of the illness. Stay focused
and aware.*

4) Remember you cannot do it all. *Give yourself permission to take
    care of your self and your illness while others help you take care of
    your children.*

What to say to your older children

My general rule of thumb with regard to talking to children about
serious adult issues is: Why tell the whole truth when the truth is
enough? This doesn't mean you should lie. Nor does it mean you
should overwhelm your child with inappropriate details. It simply
means you should adjust what you say according to the age,
developmental stage, and level of maturity of your child. You and
your husband are the best ones to determine what and how much
to say to your children. My own feeling is that younger children
should be informed that you are "sick," that you are getting help,
that you are seeing a doctor and most importantly, that you are
going to get better.

It's okay for children to know you aren't feeling well. It's much
better for children to think you are sick and getting help from a
doctor than for them to think you are just miserable and not in
the mood to be their mother right now! A young child is much
more likely to understand that you are tired and need to take a
nap than that he should stop making so much noise, get out of
the room, and leave you alone! Be honest about much of how
you are feeling while at the same time reassuring your child that
you are in good hands and will soon be back to your old self. In
the meantime, spend whatever time you feel comfortable and
capable of spending with your child, particularly during moments
you feel stronger and more positive. Grab those opportunities
and share the space with your children. If those moments are too
few and far between, then wait until you feel stronger. That's
okay, too.

How to deal with extended family, in-laws, neighbors, friends, and other well-meaning people

There's only one thing that needs to be said here. And it needs to be said over and over and over again. It's very short. It's very simple. Women who have worked with me know this very well because they hear me say it time and time again. These two short words can hold the key to a smooth recovery during PPD: *Set limits.*

If you are not already able to set limits or are not interested in getting better at establishing and maintaining appropriate boundaries, you are in for a postpartum ride that will be longer and rougher than one that is shielded by the strength of your convictions. Whether it's sleep that you need, or relief from listening to a phone ringing, or solitude from well-intended visitors, you need to get good at saying "no" when your gut feelings tell you that it's time to. The tendency to overdo and overextend during the postpartum period is widespread among new moms. It's important that you learn how to distinguish between the times you need to say YES (when others ask if they can help and your inclination is to do everything yourself!) and when to say NO (when others ask if they can come over and you're exhausted and would prefer to rest rather than entertain but are hesitant to say this because you are worried about what they will think!).

Learning when and how to set appropriate limits is not an option. It is essential to maximizing your comfort level and regaining control over how you feel.

Sometimes, one or two simple statements are all that is needed:

"I'd love to _____ but I'm not feeling up to it, maybe another time."
"This isn't a good time for me to _____. Thanks for understanding."
"I know this is hard for you to understand, but right now, I can't _____."

When setting limits, hesitation will invite scrutiny. Be clear. Be concise. Be confident. No excuses are required. No long explanations are necessary.

In summary, your postpartum experience by definition will impact others and tempt those who care for you to surround you with love, unsolicited counsel, and assorted other viewpoints. If you are depressed during your postpartum experience, this circle of sustenance can get crowded quickly. You and your husband need to be discriminating about where you go for support and from whom you accept it. While depression can cause ripple effects into your stream of support, you remain at the helm. *Do not let the symptoms that can make you feel powerless convince you that you have no power.*

Making a postpartum plan

"Watch me"

Kim sat quietly beside her husband as he bent down to gather the toys left scattered by their busy three year-old. Characteristic of those final few minutes between the end of the session and the transition out the door, we all seemed distracted by the chaos of the moment; a toddler raring to go, a check that had to be written, the "do-we-have-everything-we-came-with" moment and of course, concluding remarks and questions pertaining to the big event that lies ahead of them. Without warning, Kim blurted out, "watch me!" Her husband and I turned abruptly to make sure she was all right. "You okay?" I asked, looking closely at her face. Her eyes told me how scared she felt all of a sudden.

"I'm fine." She reassured us. "I'm fine. But watch me."

"What do you mean?" her husband asked.

"Watch me. After the baby comes, when you think everything is fine and we're so wrapped up in the excitement and the whirlwind and blinded by our euphoria, don't forget to watch me. Listen to me. Look at me. Don't forget that I might not always be the best judge of what's going on or even of how I'm feeling. I need you to do that with me, *for* me. 'Cause I might not be able to do it for myself. Okay?"

This is when it hit me. No matter how much work we have done to prepare her, no matter how many plans we have made to reassure her and strategize to protect her, no matter how many steps we taken to decrease the odds of her experiencing a recurrence of depression, she remains apprehensive.

And, it is likely true for you, too.

I can say all the right things, your husband and doctor can say all the right things, we can promise you we will do our best regardless of what unfolds, but the harsh reality persists: No one has more information and no one is better equipped to get you through this than you yourself. You are the one who carries the burden of anguish of your past experience. You are the one who needs to sort out what worked best for you and what made things worse. You are the one who knows what should be said and what exact words should be spoken. And yes, you are, more likely than not, the one who has to write the script for your husband to read if you want him to say what you know you need to hear.

Therefore, the final two worksheets may be the most important ones. The first is the **Pregnancy Support Form**: *Postpartum Plan* that we use at The Postpartum Stress Center at some point during the pregnancy, usually during the midpoint, so plans can be finalized in advance. This form is ideal for use with your therapist and doctor after completion. Sit down with your partner and fill it out together, this can begin a dialogue between the two of you that will put your expectations out in the open.

Pregnancy Support Program

Postpartum Plan

Today's date _____

    Name _____ ____wks/mos pregnant Due date ____

    Partner _____

    Address _____

    Home Phone _____

    OBGYN/midwife (name/number) _____

    Hospital _____

1. Did your mother experience PPD? Y / N don't know

2. Previous PPD or previous episode of clinical depression? Y / N don't know

3. Have you ever been treated with medication for a depressive episode? Y / N
   If yes, list medications below:

       a) _____

       b) _____

       c) _____

       d) _____

4. Problems with these medications? _____

5. Prescribing physician _____ phone _____

6. Previous therapy? Y / N If Yes, when, _____
   Comments about the experience? _____

7. How do you feel about taking medication, in general, for symptoms of depression?

       ❑ If it helps me feel and function better, it's something I
   would do

❑ I have no problems taking medication if I need it
❑ I have significant reservations about it but would consider
❑ I'd like to avoid medication if possible
❑ I have no intention of taking medication

8. During this pregnancy how are you feeling in general?:

Physically:
❑ No concerns at this time
❑ Good, normal worries related to pregnancy
❑ Not as good as I'd like
❑ Experiencing some symptoms that concern me

Emotionally:
❑ No concerns at this time
❑ Good, normal worries related to pregnancy
❑ Not as good as I'd like
❑ Experiencing some symptoms that concern me

9. Current treatment or professional support:

❑ I am seeing a therapist now *name*: _____
❑ I am seeing a psychiatrist now *name*: _____
❑ I am a member of a support group *explain*: _____
❑ I am taking antidepressant medication *explain*: _____

10. How worried are you about the postpartum period?
   1 2 3 4 5 → most worried

11. How helpful do you anticipate your partner being?
   1 2 3 4 5 → most helpful

12. Please list available support persons and *rate* the support 1 → 5
   a) _____ ____ b) _____ ____
   c) _____ ____ d) _____ ____

13. What specific concerns has your partner expressed to you, about the pregnancy, delivery, or postpartum? _____

14. What concerns do *you* have regarding *his* concerns? _____

15. Do you plan on having hired help (doula, baby nurse, housekeeper, babysitter)? Y / N / Undecided *(If doula, indicate agency and # of days per week or duration of their service)* _____
    Are there plans for family member to visit and/or assist you on a regular basis for a period of time? Y/N _____

16. Have you been evaluated during this pregnancy for medication?

       ❏ Yes, by a psychiatrist   Name _____
                                              Phone _____
       ❏ Yes, by my OBGYN   Name _____
                                              Phone _____
       ❏ No, but I plan to   Name _____
                                              Phone _____
       ❏ No, I have no plans at this time.

17. If you were successfully treated with antidepressants in the past, what is the current plan?

       ❏ I would like to start the medication in the final trimester of pregnancy.
       ❏ I will see how I feel during the course of this pregnancy and assess along the way.
       ❏ I would like to avoid taking any medication during this pregnancy even if I feel bad.
       ❏ I plan to start medication immediately upon delivery.
       ❏ I will wait and see how I feel during the postpartum period to determine whether I take medication.
       ❏ My husband and I have carefully discussed this issue of medication and we are in agreement. Y/ N If no, please describe unresolved points of discussion.

18. If you were previously or currently working outside the home what is the current plan? (Check all that apply)

    ❑ I will return to work following my scheduled leave of _____ wks / mos

    ❑ I plan to work part / full time when I return

    ❑ I plan to stay home indefinitely, depending on circumstances

    ❑ I have been given a great deal of flexibility regarding my return

    ❑ I feel I have few choices regarding my work schedule and options.

    ❑ I am still in the process of determining the plan that suits me and my family the best.

    ❑ My husband and I are not in total agreement about this plan.

    ❑ I feel quite ambivalent about my decision to work or stay home.

    ❑ I feel very comfortable with my decision to work or stay home.

    ❑ Other feelings I have regarding this choice: _____

19. What worries you most about the upcoming postpartum period?

_____

Have you discussed this concern with your partner? Y / N

If no, why not _____

If yes, what was his response? _____

20. Is there anything else you think we should know? _____

_____

The second worksheet should be kept safe under your pillow or tattooed to your chest and to your husband's body as well. Do not separate yourself from the information on this worksheet. Kim referred to it as her *I-know-you-love-me-but-since-you-don't-have-a-clue-as-to-what-to-say-to-me-when-I-feel-this-way-please-read-this* certificate. For the sake of brevity, we refer to it as your **Postpartum Pact**. Implicit in the formation of this pact is an agreement that you and your husband will go over the specifications together and discuss at length all points included particularly any that need clarification or explanation. Some of this was set in motion in the *Pregnancy as Preparation* chapter. In the Postpartum Pact, the terms will be more specific and succinct.

In some ways, this pact represents the essence of this book as well as the heart and soul of your work. It is, in most ways, a contract between you and your partner, revealing your deepest concerns as you develop your plan of action. This will augment your communication and promote a greater sense of control for both of you. Find some time when you have no distractions and you can devote total attention to reading this together and review every detail.

Our Postpartum Pact

We are reading this together because I need your help. It's possible that after the birth of our baby, I might not feel well. Since I'm at risk for depression again, we need to be alert for some of the signs so we can take care of things right away.

I need to trust that you will be observant and candid about what you see and what concerns you.

You need to trust that I am a good judge of how I am feeling.

In the event that my symptoms interfere with my ability to determine how I am feeling or what is best for me, it is crucial that you solicit help from our family, our friends, my doctor, and my therapist. We both know that it is better to be overly cautious than to assume things will get better on their own.

I need you to tell me now that you understand how important all of this is and that you are prepared to act accordingly. Knowing this will give me great comfort.

These are questions that may help you determine how things are going after our baby is born. They may not all apply to us, but they will provide a general outline for us to follow. As we review each point together, we will highlight those that feel particularly relevant to our situation so we don't miss a thing. If any feeling or experience that we went through has been overlooked, we will discuss that together and add it to the pact. After our baby comes, I will depend on you to go over these items a number of times at various stages since things can potentially change.

*   *   *

Here's what I need you to look for

- Am I acting like myself?
- Is there anything I am saying or doing that seems out of character to you or not like my usual self?
- Am I too worried, too withdrawn, too talkative, too euphoric, too exhausted, hyper, too unhappy, too uninterested?
- Do I seem confused?
- Am I crying all the time?
- Am I eating the way I usually do?
- Am I taking care of myself the way I typically do?
- Am I spending time with the baby?
- Am I reacting appropriately to the baby?
- Do I seem too worried or too detached regarding the baby?
- Am I less interested in things that used to interest me?
- Is my anxiety getting in the way of doing what I need to do?
- Do I seem preoccupied with worry or fear that seems out of proportion to you?
- Do I resist spending time with people who care about me?
- Do I seem too attentive or concerned with the baby's health?
- Am I having trouble sleeping, even when the baby is sleeping?
- Am I overly concerned with things being done perfectly with no room for mistakes?
- Are you noticing that I am isolating myself though I am fearful of being alone?
- Am I too angry, too irritable, too anxious, too short-tempered?
- Am I having panic attacks, where I say I can't breathe or think clearly?

Here's what I need you to listen for

- Am I saying anything that scares you?
- Do I say that I think something is wrong?

- Do I say I just don't feel like myself?
- Am I telling you I can't or don't want to do something that surprises you?
- Am I telling you I want leave or stop all this or hurt myself?
- Am I asking you for things I don't usually ask for?
- Am I saying I'm too scared or too tired or too unable to do what I need to do?
- Am I asking you to stay home with me all the time?
- Am I telling you I can't do this without your help?
- Am I expressing feelings of inadequacy, failure, or hopelessness?
- Do I keep asking you for reassurance or ask to you repeat the same thing over and over?
- Am I complaining a lot about how I feel physically (headaches, stomach aches, chest pains, shortness of breath)?
- Am I telling you we made a mistake and I don't want this baby?
- Am I blaming everything on our marriage?
- Am I worried that you'll leave me?
- Do I tell you that you and the baby would be better off without me?
- Am I afraid I will always feel this way?
- Do I tell you I'm a bad mother?

Here's what I need you to do

- Check in with me on a regular basis, several times a day. Ask me how I'm feeling and ask me what you can do to help.
- Enlist our friends and family to help whenever possible during the early weeks. Even if I resist, please insist that it's better for me to accept the help.
- Remind me that I've been through this before and things got better.
- Help me even if I don't ask.
- Insist that I rest even if I'm not able to sleep.
- Make sure I eat, even if I'm not hungry.

- Spend as much time caring for the baby as you can.
- If you are the slightest bit worried, encourage me to contact my doctor and therapist. If I protest, tell me that you will call them for me and come with me to the appointment. Remind me that even if everything's okay, it may be helpful and reassuring to make an appointment so we know for certain.
- Take a walk with me.
- Help with the baby during the night. If you're not able to, please make sure someone else is there to help out so I don't get sleep deprived which would make everything worse.
- Trust your instincts if you are worried or you think something needs to be done differently.
- Talk to me. Tell me what you're thinking.
- Sit with me. Stay close even when there's nothing to say.
- Help me get professional help.
- Help me find the joy. Help me stay present and appreciate the little things. Help me find and feel the butterflies, the giggles, the hugs, the sunshine, the belly laughs, the smiles.

Here's what I need you NOT to do or say

- Do not assume I am fine because I say I am.
- Do not leave everything up to me if I am feeling overwhelmed.
- Do not use this time to work harder or later or longer if I need you home during the first few weeks.
- Do not tell me to snap out of it. I can't.
- Do not let my resistance or denial get in the way of what we need to do.
- Do not tell everyone how well I'm doing if I'm not doing well.
- Please do not tell me I am strong and can do this without help if I need help.
- Please do not sabotage any effort I might need to make to seek treatment, such as resisting medication or pressuring me about the financial strain.

- Do not complain about the cost of treatment.
- Do not pressure me to have sex while I'm feeling so bad.
- Please do not do anything behind my back. If you are worried, let me know. If you want to call my doctor, let me know you are doing this.
- Do not forget to take care of yourself during this time. Make sure you are eating well, resting as much as possible, finding support for yourself from friends and family.

Here's what I need you to say

- Tell me you will do whatever I need you to do to make sure I feel healthy.
- Tell me you can tolerate my anxiety, my fears, my irritability, my moodiness.
- Tell me you are keeping an eye on how I am feeling so things won't get out of hand.
- Tell me you love me.
- Tell me I'm a good mother.
- Tell me its okay if things aren't perfect all the time.
- Tell me you are not going to leave me no matter what.

Here's what I need you to remember

- I'm doing the best I can.
- Sometimes the big things that seem scary at first aren't as scary as more subtle things. For instance, if I have an anxiety attack or snap at you, even though it's upsetting, it may not be as troublesome as if I'm isolating myself in the bedroom and quietly withdrawing.
- If you're not sure about something regarding how I am feeling or how I am acting, please ask for help and tell me you will call my doctor or therapist.
- If I become symptomatic, chances are things will not get better on their own.

- Do not underestimate how much I appreciate the fact that I
  know I can count on you during difficult times.

Things we need to add to this list

- _____
- _____
- _____
- _____
- _____
- _____

Great expectations

Despite the timeless image of the perfect pregnancy and idealized portrayals of a new mother and her baby, women with a history of postpartum depression know there is a darker side to motherhood that is sometimes ignored, sometimes sensationalized, and usually misunderstood. Let's face it, it's something many healthcare practitioners and many women and their families would prefer not to talk about. PPD falls into that category of magical thinking: *If I don't think about it, maybe it won't happen.* It doesn't work that way and even if you know that, it can still be tempting to hope it just doesn't happen again.

Nonetheless, you have decided to do something about it this time. You have taken on the task of confronting what you know to be a harsh reality, based on your own experience, and set out to reclaim a sense of control and purpose. Your ultimate undertaking will now be to remain steady in spite of what may be tenuous prospects and continue on course, supporting your efforts and believing in yourself above all.

The concept of believing in yourself is one that does not come naturally for a great many women. The temptation to strive for perfection or make comparisons to how others seem to be doing everything better is universal. These tendencies toward excellence at all costs can clash with the very real desire to find an inner peace and sense of balance.

And so, in our final stage toward reconciliation and appreciation of the work you have been through, we will consider this question:

Has there been any *meaning to the suffering* you have endured through your previous postpartum depression?

While at a party celebrating the 50th birthday of a close friend, I was introduced to a young mother who was soon due to deliver her second child. Amy told me she was looking forward to this pending delivery and was excited about her new baby coming. We chit-chatted a bit about babies and motherhood and challenges, which then led to a discussion of what she called, her "postpartum torture chamber."

"I was locked in a world I knew nothing about. I didn't know who I had become. All my feelings felt like they belonged to someone else. I couldn't function. I couldn't ask for help. I sat in a corner of my kitchen waiting for my husband to come home and rescue me. Literally, I sat on the floor, curled up in a ball, listening to my rapid breath. I tried forever to pretend like everything was okay, that this was all a bad dream that I would wake up and love my baby and say and do all the things I knew good mothers should do. But I couldn't get it together. How simple this should be, I remember thinking. Everyone does it. Everyone else can have a baby and just go on their merry way. Why was I trapped by thoughts and feelings and visions that didn't belong to me? What was happening to me?

"When Ryan was six months old, my husband came home from work and found me in that sweet corner of my kitchen. It was the first time I didn't have the strength to get up and fake it. The baby was in his high chair, I don't know for sure how long he was there, but he was crying and food was all over the place. My husband David was mortified. I still couldn't move. I remember sitting still, with my arms wrapped around my trembling knees, unable to find the strength or the motivation to get up. That's when he knew, for sure. That's when I knew this was way worse than we thought and it wasn't going to get better by itself.

"I need help," I whispered with the little breath I had left. Take me someplace. Take me now."

"Everything had been unbelievably awful until that very second when I asked for help. In a weird way, it actually felt better to tell David how bad it was, no more charades, no more wasted energy, no more faking it. At that moment, I knew I would either die or get better."

As I learned through the rest of our conversation, Amy's recovery went smoothly—as far as any recovery from a serious illness goes—she was out of the hospital in a few days, feeling less fragile and better able to cope. She continued by telling me how hopeful she was, after this traumatic experience with depression after her first baby. *Good*, I remarked, *that you're optimistic about this, that will help*. I wondered, silently, if her confidence would in fact help protect her along the way and how, after such pain, could she remain so hopeful?

"You know, it's funny," she seemed eager to continue, "I feel better about things now that I've been through all of that. I mean, don't get me wrong, it was horrible at the time, but I know, for many reasons, I'm better off now after going through it."

While she finished recalling her story, I was intrigued by the smile on her face, the loving words she chose when she spoke of her husband, and the heartfelt wish for an uneventful postpartum period this next time. I started thinking about what, if any, valuable lessons could come from such an unsettling time in their young relationship. Furthermore, why are some couples better able to unite in this effort and emerge even stronger while others are swept away by the turbulence? The simple answer, though more simple to say than to realize, is to maintain a positive attitude so lessons can be learned and personal growth can occur.

Social scientists have long claimed that there are definite characteristics associated with positive adaptation. These characteristics can be difficult to switch on and off and are more personality features than things you can decide to do or not do at a given moment. In other words, if you're prone to be a worrier, it's hard to just stop worrying because you know you "should" or because people tell you you'll feel better if you do. But if it's true that people with a more positive mind-set are better able to cope and heal faster, it makes sense that we should at least *try* to improve our outlook in search of meaning and the potential for growth. We should do this, partly because common sense tells us this is right, partly because we know it helps people recover faster and mostly because, truthfully, it feels better.

Some of the characteristics that have been linked with positive adjustment potential are: (Taylor, S.E. 1983)

- Positive reinterpretation of stressful events (reframing)
- Active coping and planning
- Seeking social support and making connections
- Humor
- Ability to accept and trust current state of being
- Rearranging priorities and making compromises
- Insight and self-expression
- Capacity for or interest in intimacy
- Spiritual connections or pursuit

Take a look at above list and try to determine how many of these characteristics you possess or on which you can improve. When we look more closely at these traits we can begin to understand how they relate to emotional and physical resilience. Resilience in this context refers to your ability to successfully adapt to stressful life events. Being flexible in the face of stressors is never easy. It requires the interplay between your attitudes, your beliefs, your behavior, your feelings, your environment, and how you view the world.

Resilience can be learned. It's hard, particularly if it's not your default disposition or if you're naturally a negative thinker. But it's worth working on. Anytime you make the effort to deliberately change your thinking like this, it's tough. It's like building a muscle you haven't used before. Imagine lifting an 8-lb dumbbell up and down to strengthen your biceps. It's hard the first time. You have to keep up the repetitions and maintain the workout schedule for a while before you see the results of your efforts. Remind yourself that that it's the same thing when you are learning how to embrace a new way of thinking. It's hard. It might not feel natural for you. But if you practice saying the right words, whether you believe them or not at this point, you might discover that the rewards, in the long run, are huge.

Tips to help foster resilience during the postpartum period:

- Understand and accept that there will be changes and disappointments.
- Understand and accept that some things will be out of your control.
- Reach out and establish or maintain important connections.
- Set small achievable goals for yourself. Be realistic about how much you can or should expect yourself to do.
- Set forth active coping strategies. Make a plan, expect it to change, make another plan. Take action, don't wait for things to change.
- Pay attention to personal needs and feelings. Be particularly mindful of what makes you feel good.
- Ask for and accept assistance from others.
- Look for laughs, hugs, giggles and fun in the most unlikely places.
- Maintain positive thinking. Try to focus on how you'd like things to be rather than how worried you might feel.
- Find quiet time. Breathe.

This process you are going through will provide you with invaluable resources. As you continue to search for meaning and understanding from lessons learned, you will gain a sense of mastery. This comes from feeling more in control of the situation. *What can be done differently? How can I behave in ways that may change the way I feel?* These are examples of the cognitive strategies you are developing that will maximize personal control and minimize your feelings of helplessness.

In conclusion, the work you have done here is quite a testament to your commitment to taking care of yourself. As you look forward, brace for the unknown, prepare for many possibilities, and expect the worst to some extent—it's no wonder you feel anxious about what lies ahead. This anxiety, as unwelcome as it may feel at first, will act as a vital catalyst to this process. If you had no anxiety about the potential risks, you might avoid doing the work or taking the steps necessary to protect yourself sufficiently. Accept this level of anxiety and proceed in spite of it, taking it right along side of you throughout the process. Remember that you can be in control and feel anxious at the same time.

As you continue in the direction that your heart leads you, remember to check in every so often with your partner. Are you both on the same page? Does he have all the same information you have? Are the two of you sharing this journey? Do not make the mistake of assuming things will take care of themselves. Keep your eyes and heart open to everything around you. Be smart. Stay on top of how you are feeling and what needs to be done. Be your own best advocate. Ask for help when you need it. Do not cast blame on yourself or anyone else if things get off course. Stay focused. Breathe deeply. Above all, believe in your self and the choices you make. It will be okay.

Appendix I

From a husband who's been there and back and there again . . .

I never thought that we would ever be at a point where Amy would tell me that she was that sad, that things seemed so hopeless that she really didn't see the point in going on any further. Just a few days earlier, things had seemed to be on the upswing. But here we were. It was surreal—here was a woman I knew and loved, who wanted nothing more than to have and raise children, and the idea of having another baby absolutely sickened her. The joy of our life, our 2-year old son, did nothing but annoy her. This was so clearly a chemical phenomenon—one minute she would be pretty close to the Amy I knew, the next she would be almost unrecognizable, with barely a flicker of the light in her eye which had made me ask her to marry me. A roller coaster ride, indeed—if it wasn't so serious. But this was still her, and we needed help. Sure, I thought I had done a decent job of letting her know how much I loved her, how great I thought she was, and I had tried to help her with the day to day parenting responsibilities as much as I could. And she had been speaking with Karen for some time now. But once she started talking about hurting herself, I was out of my league. We called Karen immediately, and Amy got better—much more slowly than immediately. Therapy, medication, and love. A long, tiring, but ultimately rewarding journey, which we have yet to complete. Advice from the front lines:

Plan on the long haul. Sure, there is an inclination to think that your wife will be different, that this problem will be gone in no time. But that is simply not a reasonable expectation, so disabuse yourself (and your wife) of the notion, as such thinking can only have negative consequences. You and your wife NEED to be realistic about what you're facing.

Have a support group. If you have family in the area, use them! Make sure someone is around to check in on your wife when you're at work, and make sure she knows whom she should call if she needs something and you're not immediately available. If there is no family around, friends and neighbors will do, so long as your wife can get comfortable with them. On a related note, try not to let feelings of embarrassment get in the way of obtaining the help that you and your wife need. This can be difficult if your wife (like mine) is proud and doesn't want to let people know she is struggling. Try to convince her (gently!) that this thing is just too big to let pride interfere with getting the necessary help. Everyone needs help at some point in their lives—this is her time!

Get professional help! This is a medical condition which, frighteningly, can be a life or death situation. Find the money and spend it, just as you would if your wife needed a lung transplant. Some wives will need convincing that they even need help—try to help them see otherwise.

Tell her that you love her, that you are going to help her through this, and that you really don't care how long it takes. If you start to feel hopeless yourself (which will probably happen at least once), try not to let her see it. See if you can get away for a couple hours to recharge your batteries.

She is not a failure or a wimp. She is a human being, and by design, human beings are not perfect. If it were any other way, the concept of "help" would not exist. This is why you are here, this is why you married her—to help her when she needs it. Tell her this! Remind her that when you need it, you plan on having her repay the favor.

Know that it stinks. Believe the experts when they describe the nightmare your wife is going through. Try to make her understand this as well. But you can turn this around a bit and let her know that, while it may seem absolutely impossible, what is happening to her is normal, and at some point it ends.

If there is a child around, try to pay attention to his or her needs and reactions. Your children's perceptions are much better than you would believe, and it is all too easy to forget about them in the midst of trying to deal with this situation.

A whole bunch of work? Yes. But should you be faced with the situation, remember always that it can be done. And believe it or not, there can be silver linings. This is your moment to show your wife, and yourself, what being her husband means to you.

References

Beck CT, Reynolds MA, Rutowski P Maternity blues and postpartum depression *J Obstet Gyneco* 1992: 21(4):287-293.

Cooper PJ, Murray L Prediction, detection and treatment of postnatal depression. *Arch Dis Child* 1997; 77:97-99.

Edhborg M, Seimyr L, Lundh W, Widstroem A: The long-term impact of postnatal depression mood on the mother-child interaction. Karolinska Institute, Stockholm, Sweden 2000

Hale, T Medications and mothers milk, 7th edition Amarillo, Pharmasoft 1998-99.

Lawrence, R Breastfeeding: A guide for the medical profession, 5th ed. St Louis: Mosby 1999.

Murray, L., Fiori-Cowley, A., Hooper, R., Cooper, P: The impact of postnatal depression and associated adversity on early mother-infant interactions and later infant outcome. *Child Development* 1996 *67*, 2512-2526.

Nunocs, R, Cohen, L, Viguera A, Reminick A, Harlow B: Risk for recurrent depression during the postpartum period: A prospective study. Massachusetts General Hospital & Harvard Medical School, Boston MA.

Pitt B, 1973 Maternity blues. *Br J Psychiatry* 1973;122:431-3.

Spencer J: Medications in the breastfeeding mother. *Am Fam Physician* 2001.

Stowe, ZN, Nemeroff CB: Women at risk for postpartum onset major depression. *Am J Obstet Gynecol* 1995. August 173 (2): 639-45.

Stowe ZN, Owens MJ, Landry JC, Kilts C, Ely T., Llewellyn A, Nemeroff C.B. Sertraline and desmethylsertraline in human breast milk and nursing infants. *American Journal of Psychiatry* 1997 154:1255-1260.

Wisner KL, Parry BL, and Pointek CM. Postpartum depression: *N Engl J Med* 2002 347(3); 194-199.

Wisner, KL, Peindl KS, Gigliotti T: Obsessions and compulsions in women with postpartum depression. *J Clin Psychiatry* 1999 March, 60 (3):176-80.

Wisner KL, Perel JM, Findling RL: Antidepressant treatment during breast-feeding. Am J Psychiatry 1996 153(9): 1132-1137.

CPSIA information can be obtained at www.ICGtesting.com
Printed in the USA
LVOW08s1721130816

500262LV00001B/70/P